ROTARY INTERNATIONAL®

CONQUERING POLIO

A brief history of PolioPlus, Rotary's role in a global program
to eradicate the world's greatest crippling disease

HERBERT A. PIGMAN

ISBN 0-915062-28-3

Cover photo: Jean-Marc Giboux
Cover and interior design: Reiko Takahashi

CONTENTS

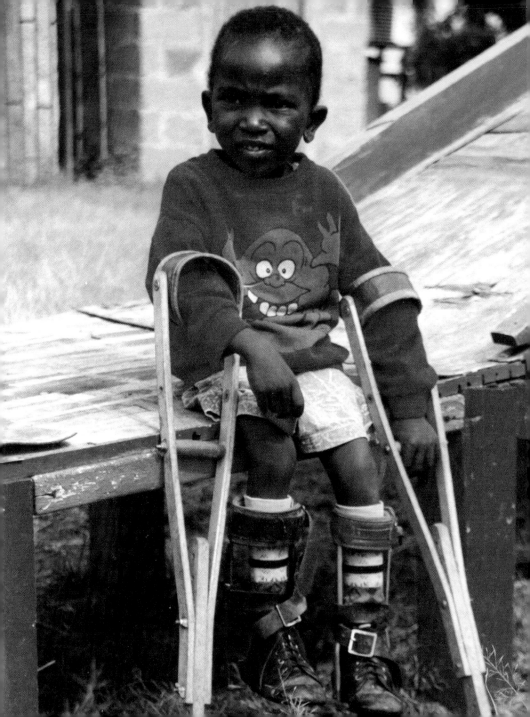

PREFACE

Rotary's war on polio began in 1979 with a commitment to buy and help deliver vaccine to six million children in the Philippines. It was the first project conceived under Rotary's new Health, Hunger and Humanity (3-H) program and a test of Rotarians' capacity to serve effectively, on a massive scale, in the field of public health. Its success spurred the planning of the most ambitious program in Rotary's 75-year history: the immunization of all the world's children against polio.

Campaigns were undertaken in other countries in the next five years. By 1985, with the advice and support of Dr. Albert Sabin, developer of the oral polio vaccine, Rotary had forged a global strategy: establish partnerships with health agencies and national health ministries, raise money to buy vaccine, and enlist the one million Rotary club members as foot soldiers in the task of delivering the vaccine to the more than 100 million children born each year in developing countries. The name of the program, PolioPlus, embraced both the quest for a polio-free world and the belief that an attack targeting polio would also help to raise immunization levels against five other childhood infectious diseases that were killing and disabling millions of children each year.

Buoyed by the success of polio immunization campaigns, particularly in the Americas under the leadership of the Pan American Health Organization,

Opposite: Polio was killing or paralyzing 1,000 people a day when in 1985 Rotary launched its PolioPlus program and pledged to immunize all the world's children against the dreaded disease. A few cents' worth of vaccine provides lifetime immunity.

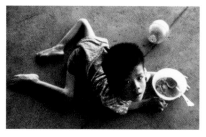

on 12 May 1988 the 166 nations of the World Health Assembly unanimously resolved to eradicate polio. At the time, the poliovirus was circulating in 125 countries, paralyzing or killing 1,000 people a day, mostly children. In the next 12 years, despite problems of funding, civil strife, war, weak health infrastructures, and impoverished national economies, Rotary and its spearheading partners, the World Health Organization, UNICEF, and the U.S. Centers for Disease Control and Prevention, made spectacular progress. Almost two billion children had received oral polio vaccine. As the 20th century drew to a close, only 20 countries remained polio endemic.

Since then, the noose has been drawn ever tighter on the poliovirus, the world's greatest crippler. Certification of the eradication of the virus will require a minimum of three years of zero polio cases following the discovery of the last case of polio. During this period, countries must maintain intensive surveillance as well as sufficiently high levels of immunization of their newborn populations.

This brief history is published in celebration of Rotary's 100th anniversary, as the world girds itself for the final battles in the war on polio. It is dedicated to the thousands of Rotary leaders, Rotarians, friends, RI staff members, and professional colleagues in partner agencies (far too numerous to list) who have shared generously of their time, treasures, and talents to ensure that precious drops of polio vaccine reach every child in even the poorest and most remote villages of the world. For the past 25 years, they have kept the dream alive. The eradication of polio, the most terrifying of all crippling diseases, will be the monument to their work.

H.A.P.

June 2004

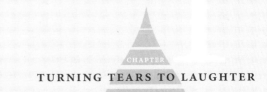

TURNING TEARS TO LAUGHTER

TURNING TEARS TO LAUGHTER

O N NEW YEAR'S Day in 1986, Rotary publicly announced to a global audience that it had embarked on the most ambitious humanitarian program in the service organization's 80-year history: the immunization of all the world's children against polio.

The occasion for the announcement was the famed Rose Parade in Pasadena, California, USA, part of the annual Tournament of Roses, in which scores of floats bedecked with flowers flow past thousands of people. Cameras telecast the spectacle to 125 million viewers in the United States and around the world.

Rotary's parade entry was neither the largest nor most expensive of the more than 100 units in the 1986 Rose Parade. But no float surpassed it in terms of the response it evoked among viewers. They saw and spontaneously acclaimed its message: Rotary was launching an all-out, global war on the dreaded disease of poliomyelitis, a disease that was then killing or crippling 1,000 people a day. "Good luck, Rotary!" "Keep up the good work!" cheered spectators along the parade route.

The float depicted an abandoned wheelchair, symbolic of Rotary's quest for a world in which no child would be disabled by polio. Rotary Youth Exchange students in national dress danced around a tree set in a garden of flowers. Atop the tree flew a banner bearing the date 2005, the centennial year of Rotary's founding as well as the target date for a polio-free world. A "Stop Polio" symbol, a red circle with a diagonal slash across the word *polio,* symbolized the float's theme, Turning Tears to Laughter.

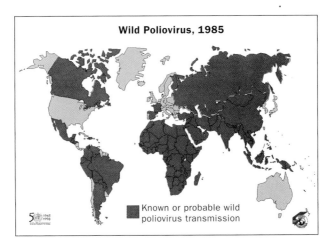

Undaunted by the global reach of the disease, Rotary became the world's leading private-sector partner in the eradication of poliomyelitis. By the time the world is certified polio-free, Rotary will have committed more than $600 million plus an army of volunteers, helping to bring oral polio vaccine to more than two billion children.

The dream of a polio-free world caught the imagination of millions that morning. But only a few knew the story behind the courageous, young African man who was riding aboard the float. On legs paralyzed by polio but supported by braces, he stood throughout the three-hour parade, smiling and waving, acknowledging the cheers of the crowd and thanking Rotary for giving him a new lease on life.

Twenty years earlier, 12-month-old Wilborn Chuvala had been infected with polio as the virus swept through the town of Karonga, Malawi, in

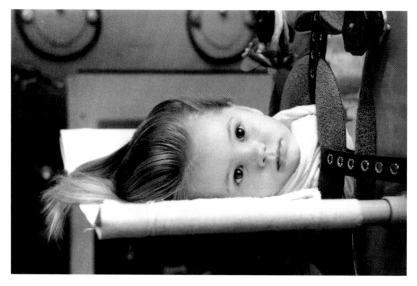

When polio paralyzes breathing muscles, the patient is placed in a so-called iron lung, a metal cylinder where alternating air pressure forces air to and from the lungs. Some polio survivors have lived months or years in iron lungs.

southern Africa. The child, who was just learning to walk, was left paralyzed from the waist down. For the next 14 years, Wilborn endured life as a "crawler," able to move about only on calloused hands and knees.

In 1981 his uncle read about an orthopedic clinic and rehabilitation center in the capital, Lilongwe, and urged his nephew to go. With a small bag of food and US$15 given to him by his uncle, the 15-year-old set out alone for the clinic, 270 miles away, traveling first by boat and bus, then by crawling and hitchhiking. Once there, Wilborn came under the care of

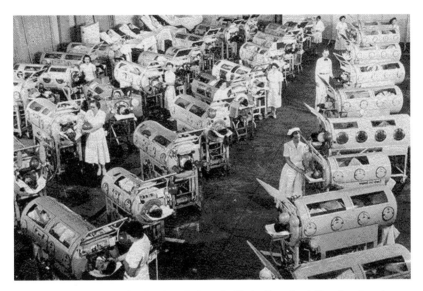

At the height of polio epidemics, hospital wards filled with polio victims for whom iron lungs provided the breath of life. Communities frequently closed schools, theaters, and swimming pools in an effort to stop the spread of the highly contagious poliovirus.

Rotarians who were sharing their surgical skills as volunteers with Rotary's Health, Hunger and Humanity (3-H) program. Among them was Dr. Joseph Serra, of Stockton, California, USA, a 50-year-old orthopedic surgeon. Serra operated on Wilborn's knees and hip and extended his Achilles tendons, enabling the teenager to stand upright, supported by braces, for the first time in his life. Wilborn later wrote to Serra: "You will be so pleased, as am I, that I walk without a crutch. I walk with a cane now. I walk like a gentleman."

Anticipating the public announcement of its polio immunization program, Rotary invited Wilborn Chuvala to travel to Pasadena and ride on Rotary's parade float. With help from British Airways, Wilborn made the long flight from Malawi to California, there to symbolize the hope that this global program of polio immunization would spare millions of children with disabilities such as his.

Serra, whose friendship with Wilborn had grown during each of his six volunteer tours of duty at the Lilongwe clinic, rode with the young man on the float. Joe and his wife, Dorothy, funded Wilborn's high school and college training. Today, the young man teaches mathematics and English in Karonga. He is married and has two children, who are named, not surprisingly, Joe and Dorothy.

Wilborn Chuvala is one of more than 10 million people who today struggle with the effects of polio, historically the world's greatest cause of disability. Before the discovery of polio vaccines, polio killed or paralyzed 600,000 people, mostly children, each year. Wilborn's experience is one of both triumph and tragedy: triumph in that his will to surmount enormous obstacles to become a contributing member of society, tragedy in that he and millions of other polio victims during the past half century would have been spared death or disability if the world's health systems had been able to deliver a few drops of vaccine, vaccine that costs only pennies a dose.

On that New Year's Day in 1986, Rotary's commitment was clear, hopes were high, and resolve was growing. Brilliant scientific work had created polio vaccines, giving health providers the basic tools needed to interrupt the transmission of the poliovirus. Only a few months earlier, the success of new strategies in the Americas had led the Pan American Health Organization to adopt a goal of polio eradication for the entire Western Hemisphere. Rotarians

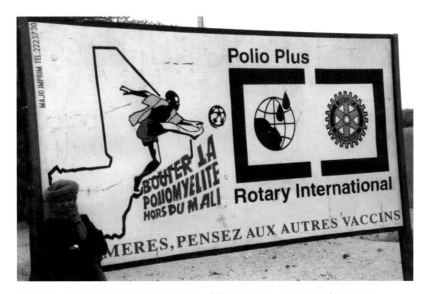

Although polio immunization is the focus of PolioPlus, the *plus* part of the name recognizes that the program also boosts efforts to immunize children against other infectious diseases such as measles, pertussis, and tetanus.

had successfully forged new program policies that had opened the door to cooperative action on a global scale. The goal seemed entirely reasonable: Marshal financial resources, create partnerships, and harness the business know-how and volunteer muscle of Rotarians to public health systems worldwide to deliver oral polio vaccine to every child, everywhere, and at the right time. Achieve this and the wild poliovirus would disappear.

The new program was named PolioPlus: *polio* to signify the program's principal focus and *plus* to express Rotary's conviction that a targeted attack on polio would also help to achieve the broader objective of raising immunization rates against other infectious diseases in developing countries, where each year 100 million children were born and millions were dying because of desperately low levels of immunization.

Although the goal was clear, no one could have anticipated the full extent of the task that lay before Rotary and its partners over the next 20 years in their quest for a polio-free world. Rotary faced the twin challenges of conducting a fundraising effort unprecedented in scope and a massive educational program to build the support of its members. Among leaders in public health, the program sparked debate about competing approaches to combating vaccine-preventable diseases. Program planners faced the enormous challenge of informing millions of parents, many with little or no previous contact with health providers, about the value of immunization. For virologists and epidemiologists, the creation of a global laboratory network was essential to a surveillance system on which success depended.

Added to these challenges, and only dimly foreseen, were the setbacks that would result from wars, economic downturns, and the continuing frailty and even collapse of public health infrastructures in some countries. And already beginning to darken the horizon were newly emerging, high-burden diseases — most notably, HIV/AIDS and multidrug-resistant tuberculosis and malaria — that were to compete for public health resources.

Clearly, if polio was to become, after smallpox, the second disease to be eradicated from the planet, these challenges had to be met.

CHAPTER 2

THE WORLD'S GREATEST CRIPPLER

THE WORLD'S GREATEST CRIPPLER

T HE EARLIEST RECORDED evidence of polio was carved in stone some 35 centuries ago on an Egyptian stele. It depicts a young man with a withered leg and a drop foot, leaning on a crutch. Paralysis of one or more limbs, with subsequent atrophy of the muscles, is a common result of poliomyelitis, an acute infectious disease caused by one of three types of poliovirus.

Poliovirus enters the body through the mouth. Close human contact, poor hygiene, and an environment in which food and water are contaminated by human feces carrying the virus are the most common avenues of poliovirus transmission. After incubation in the throat and intestines, the virus can enter the bloodstream. Unless blocked by sufficient antibodies, such as those provided by polio vaccine, the virus can invade the central nervous system, damaging or destroying those motor neurons in the spinal cord or brain stem whose function is to transmit signals to muscles of the body.

The result of such damage is sudden onset of paralysis, either of the arms, legs, or both, called acute flaccid (floppy) paralysis, or AFP. Other victims suffer paralysis of muscles that enable the functions of breathing, swallowing, and speaking, known as bulbar polio. Such victims frequently are encased from the neck down in an iron lung, a metal cylinder equipped with mechanical devices in which rhythmic alternations of air pressure force air in and out of the lungs. Many such victims regain the ability to breathe unaided, but some live for years cocooned in an iron lung or other types of artificial respirators. Historically, of every 10 people paralyzed by polio, roughly 1 will

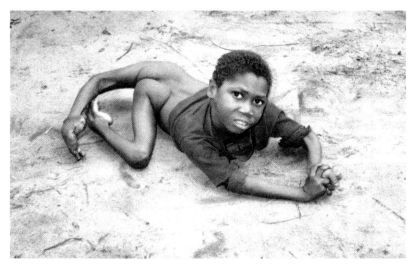

Worldwide, an estimated 10-20 million people suffer irreversible paralysis or disablement as the result of polio, making the disease the world's greatest crippler.

die, 2-3 will suffer permanent paralysis, and the remainder will recover normal functions.

For centuries, polio was an endemic disease. Under then-prevailing sanitation and hygienic conditions, most infants were exposed to and built immunity to the poliovirus while still protected by polio antibodies transmitted from their mothers. The polio epidemics that began late in the 1800s and mushroomed in the first half of the 20th century were, ironically, exacerbated by improved sanitation, particularly the installation of clean water and sewage disposal systems in urban areas.

Under these improved hygiene conditions, substantial numbers of children grew to adulthood with no exposure, and thus no immunity, to the poliovirus. When the virus invaded such vulnerable populations, it swept in without warning and with terrifying speed. Fear gripped communities. A young girl could one day be roller-skating and the next morning be racked with fever and intense pain and unable to move her legs. Schools and theaters, camps and swimming pools were shut down. Public gatherings were curtailed. Panicked parents sequestered kids at home, and some even stuffed rags in the crevices of windows and doors to hold the virus at bay. As late as 1952, almost 58,000 cases of polio were reported in the United States alone, part of the 600,000 or more cases estimated to have occurred worldwide that year.

The poliovirus is capriciously selective. Fewer than 1 percent of those infected become paralyzed. Thus, for every apparent polio-infected person, there can be in close proximity 200 or more other infected people who unknowingly are carrying and spreading the virus. Mild and short-lived polio symptoms such as fever, malaise, drowsiness, nausea, vomiting, and sore throat can go unrecognized and are often ascribed to other illnesses. Thus the poliovirus is a silent and stealthy crippler. It respects no boundaries. And whether circulating in a remote and primitive village, a region, or a mobile world society, the characteristics of the virus immensely complicate efforts to eradicate it.

Eradication has been hailed as the ultimate form of communicable-disease control, but all health experts agree that its achievement is far from easy. The possibility of eradicating any disease first emerged in 1796 when Edward Jenner, an English country physician, demonstrated that a mild infection from cowpox provided immunity against smallpox. This loathsome disease killed millions every year and often blinded or disfigured survivors.

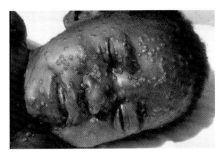

In October 1979, the World Health Organization confirmed the eradication of smallpox. It is the only disease thus far eradicated.

In the royal court of England, rare was the face that was not scarred by smallpox. Jenner observed that many milkmaids of Gloucestershire, however, had fair complexions; somehow, they had acquired immunity from smallpox. He then began his experiment to extract material from pustules on the udders of infected cows in order to vaccinate (derived from the Latin *vacca*, "cow") his patients.

Within four years, an estimated 100,000 people had been vaccinated by Jenner's method. "It now becomes too manifest to admit of controversy," Jenner wrote, "that the annihilation of smallpox, the most dreadful scourge of the human species, must be the final result of this practice." Jenner's dream was destined to become reality more than 200 years later. A concerted smallpox-eradication program was launched by the World Health Organization in 1967. At the time, there were an estimated 10-15 million cases in 44 countries. Despite the enormity of the task, the nature of smallpox gave cause for optimism: the smallpox virus, like the poliovirus, has no known reservoir other than humans. An effective vaccine was available, and a strategy of mass immunization aided by intense surveillance and containment succeeded. In October 1979, after two years of intensive search for any remaining case, WHO confirmed the eradication of smallpox.

Although the smallpox program succeeded, attempts to eradicate other diseases have failed. Among these efforts was a malaria eradication program launched in 1955 by WHO. Its success hinged on the spraying of dichloro-diphenyltrichloroethane, or DDT, an insecticide used in controlling mosquitoes, the vector for the disease. Nature decreed otherwise. The mosquito developed resistance to DDT, and the campaign failed after an expenditure of some $2 billion by WHO and other international agencies. A program to eliminate yaws, a disease that causes deforming and incapacitating lesions and can be cured by a single injection of penicillin, succeeded in only a few of the 49 countries where it operated over a 20-year period. Yellow-fever eradication efforts succumbed to the discovery of a nonhuman reservoir in monkeys.

The need to thoroughly understand the natural history of the disease was just one of the lessons learned from past attempts at eradication. The strategy to eradicate polio drew heavily upon such lessons: Initiate surveillance systems early and use the information to guide strategy and tactics, gain commitments from all political levels, coordinate donor support, set specific target dates, and develop a vertical approach that both complements and strengthens sustainable primary health services.

The key to the eradication of the poliovirus, of course, was the development of an effective oral polio vaccine. It opened the door to Rotary's PolioPlus program because it enabled massive numbers of volunteers to administer the vaccine to children, each dose consisting of two drops of vaccine squeezed into the child's mouth.

Two polio vaccines are available, and both are effective against all three types of poliovirus. An inactivated (killed) injectable polio vaccine (IPV) was developed in 1955 by Dr. Jonas Salk. A few years later, Dr. Albert Sabin succeeded in developing a live attenuated (weakened) oral polio vaccine (OPV) in his laboratories in Cincinnati, Ohio, USA, where he was a member of the Rotary Club of Cincinnati.

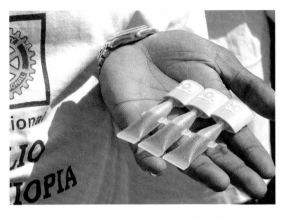

Oral polio vaccine's low cost and ease of administration by volunteers spurred WHO's decision to launch a global eradication program. Each dose costs about 10 cents. *Photo by Jean-Marc Giboux*

For purposes of eradication, oral polio vaccine became WHO's vaccine of choice. OPV does not have to be administered by trained health workers, requires no sterile needles or syringes, and at $0.10 or less a dose, is less than one-fifth the cost of IPV. In addition to protecting the individual, the oral polio vaccine also limits the multiplication of the wild (naturally occurring) virus inside the intestines, thus reducing fecal excretion of the wild virus. The shedding of polio vaccine virus in the stools of recently immunized children has a beneficial effect in poor sanitary environments in which the polio vaccine virus is spread to nonimmunized children through the oral-fecal route. This passive, or secondary, form of immunization proved to be an important additional advantage of OPV. The downside of oral polio vaccine is its ability to cause paralysis in either the vaccinated child or a close contact. A study by the U.S. Centers for Disease Control (now known as the U.S. Centers for Disease Control and Prevention, or CDC) covering an 11-year period concluded that OPV produced one case of paralysis for every 2.5 million doses administered. For several polio-free countries, the risk of OPV-related paralysis was to become too high, and they switched to IPV or a combination of the two vaccines.

The existence of an effective vaccine for polio eradication and the disappearance of smallpox were persuasive factors driving a series of decisions and actions by Rotary's leadership that led to the formal establishment of the PolioPlus program in 1985. Few of these leaders realized the ramifications of the program on which they were about to embark. And few, if any, could dream that Rotary, a private-sector organization with no track record in the field of public health, would shortly become the private-sector leader in the greatest public health adventure in history. What these leaders did share, however, was a dream of a polio-free world, a dream coupled with faith that their fellow Rotarians would put their shoulders behind the wheel of Rotary's first worldwide service program.

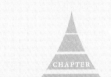

CHAPTER 3

THE SEED IS PLANTED

THE SEED IS PLANTED

POLIOPLUS WOULD NOT have been possible without the benefit of a sea change in Rotary's program policies.

For more than a half century, Rotary International had vigorously discouraged any form of corporate action intended to orchestrate local, national, regional, or global service activities for Rotary clubs. This policy derived from Resolution 23-34, adopted by the 1923 RI Convention, in St. Louis, Missouri, USA. It stated that each Rotary club had absolute autonomy in the selection of its activities and that Rotary International "should never prescribe nor proscribe any objective activity for any club."

Through the years, these principles became a mantra for Rotarians who believed that Rotary club members, individually applying the ideal of service in their everyday vocational and community affairs, best expressed the "true spirit of Rotary" as conceived by Rotary's founder, Paul Harris. In the opinion of other Rotarians, Resolution 23-34 shackled the tremendous potential of Rotary's global membership to tackle human needs beyond the capacity of any individual, club, or group of clubs.

Ironically, Resolution 23-34 was adopted in order to thwart a proposal to commit Rotary International to a formal program for the care and rehabilitation of crippled children. Since 1919, such a movement had gained substantial support in the United States. Rotary clubs had taken the lead in providing rehabilitation services and mainstreaming disabled children. But many Rotary leaders reacted negatively to crippled-children advocates' aggressive use of RI's program and administrative network. Although lauding the objective of the societies for crippled children, they feared that the tail was beginning to wag the dog. They also feared that Rotary might become one-dimensional in community service. When confronted with a proposal seeking to raise per capita dues specifically to fund a program for disabled children, Rotary International's leaders countered with Resolution 23-34. Its passage resolved problems about relationships between Rotary International and crippled-children societies, as well as other organizations. Acting independently, Rotarians continued their support of the disabled. Soon, the movement picked up additional supporters and became the National Society for Crippled Children (known today as Easter Seals).

Resolution 23-34's influence — some say stranglehold — on Rotary's policy proscribing activities initiated by Rotary International continued long after 1923. It began to erode 40 years later in 1963-64 when RI President Carl P. Miller, a *Wall Street Journal* newspaper executive, developed a program to pair arbitrarily all Rotary districts and clubs. The Matched District and Club Program was both praised and criticized, but all agreed that its purpose — to dramatically increase contact between Rotary clubs in different countries — succeeded. Meaningful Rotary contacts across national boundaries were greatly accelerated. Clubs in affluent countries began to help clubs in developing countries with projects such as drilling village wells. A club that set out to collect coins for a new propeller for a flying doctor service in Africa delivered an entire new aircraft. The number of individual Rotarians and groups visiting overseas exploded. Joint service projects increased exponentially. Soon, Rotary International became a clearinghouse for cooperative service projects. Thus Rotary's World Community Service

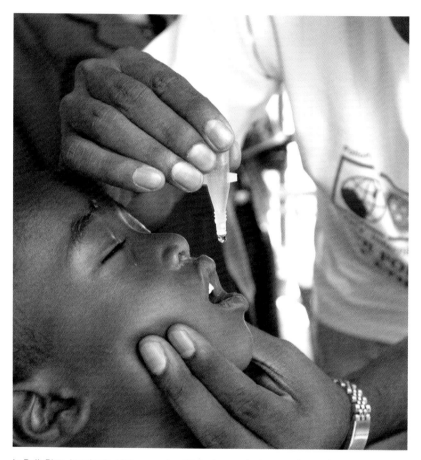

In PolioPlus, hundreds of thousands of Rotarians volunteer to give oral polio vaccine to children, mainly on National Immunization Days.
Photo by Jean-Marc Giboux

program was born. A sleeping giant had been awakened. Today, hundreds of clubs continue to establish partnerships in community projects that improve lives and meet human needs.

The growing success and popularity of World Community Service created a positive climate for RI President-elect Clem Renouf to introduce his plans for the Health, Hunger and Humanity (3-H) program. The opportunity came in February 1978 in a meeting of the RI Board of Directors. RI President Jack Davis had invited Dr. Robert Hingson, a Rotarian, to make a presentation to the Board about the benefits of immunizing children against communicable diseases. Dramatically wielding his injectable-vaccine gun, he painted a vision of how Rotary's vast network of business and professional members could help prevent the deaths of millions of children.

The next day, in response to a request that he share his plans for his year as president, Renouf expanded on this vision of Rotary's service potential by outlining a program to address human needs too large for any individual club or district to undertake and, in the process, engage Rotarians who would volunteer their vocational and professional skills in communities abroad. "As an organization," Renouf said, "we need to be recognized worldwide as one which is concerned about people and their needs, and we need to express that concern in concrete, visible, and significant programs at home and abroad. This is critical, not only to our continued growth but to our very survival in many countries of the world."

That Rotarians stood ready and willing to do this had already been demonstrated in a program known as FAIM (Fourth Avenue in Motion), in which Australian Rotarians volunteered to carry out community service projects in New Guinea and other places. Further evidence had been provided in 1963 by RI's Small Business Clinic, a pilot program in which Rotarians crossed national borders to share their business know-how with small-business owners in Colombia, Ecuador, Ghana, India, Pakistan, and the Philippines. RI leaders, however, abruptly stopped the program, ostensibly because the creation of the International Executive Service Corps, a nonprofit organization that worked in partnership with the U.S. Agency for International Development (USAID), nullified the need for Rotary's leadership in this area. In fact, Resolution 23-34 was still casting its shadow.

The 3-H program required central funding. Renouf proposed an appeal for voluntary contributions to a special fund, in honor of Rotary's 75th anniversary in 1980. Plans for this appeal met strenuous objections from the Trustees of The Rotary Foundation of RI. They feared derailment of Rotarians' growing financial support of Foundation programs. The controversy was resolved by negotiation leading to an agreement about the respective roles of the Board of Directors and the Trustees. They agreed to place the funding and administration of the 3-H program in The Rotary Foundation. In time, fears about a diminution of support for The Rotary Foundation proved to be unfounded. The 3-H program, in fact, spurred interest in international service in general and with it a growing awareness and appreciation of Foundation objectives. Financial support for all Foundation programs began a steady climb.

Based on Renouf's description of 3-H objectives at the 1978 International Assembly and RI Convention, in Tokyo, money began to flow to the 75th Anniversary Fund, eventually reaching $7.2 million. Rotarians lined up to volunteer for service abroad. And they were soon asking: Just how will the 3-H funds be used?

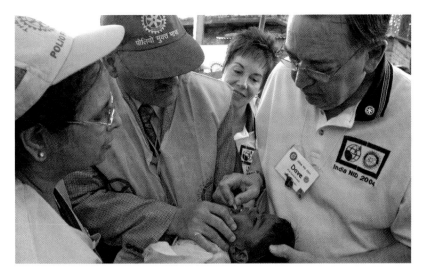

Hundreds of Rotarians from polio-free countries, such as Dave Groner (right), have traveled voluntarily to polio-endemic countries to immunize children, share fellowship with local Rotarians, and help fight the battle against polio.
Photo by Jean-Marc Giboux

The task of refining a statement of 3-H program purpose, establishing its policies and operating procedures, and communicating these to Rotary leaders at global and district levels fell to a 48-member committee representing 18 nations. Three cochairs — Dr. Ben Saltzman (health), Webster Pendergrass (hunger), and Cliff Dochterman (humanity) — met in July 1978 to draft the blueprint. From this meeting emerged a stated objective for health: "to prevent or reduce disability and to improve the mental and physical well-being of people."

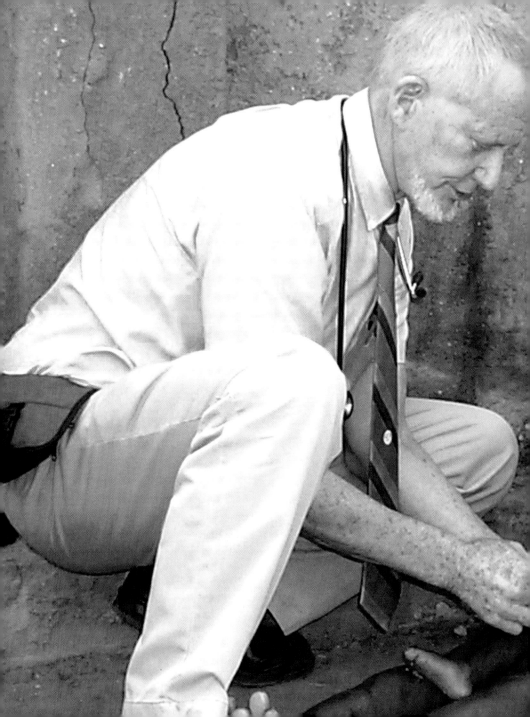

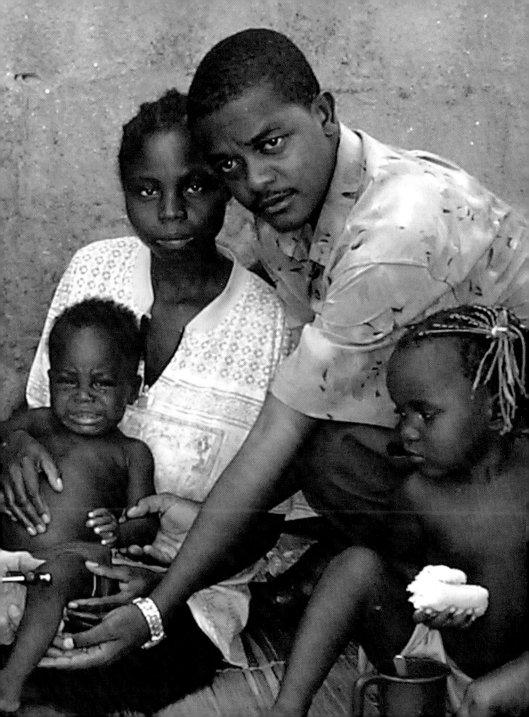

At its next meeting, in February 1979, responding to a proposal by Past District Governor Benny Santos, the 3-H Committee agreed to pursue the feasibility of a $760,000 project to buy and help distribute polio vaccine to 6.3 million children in the Philippines, a country that had one of the highest rates of polio cases in the WHO Western Pacific region. In March, Renouf, Santos, and others met with the Philippine minister of health, who approved Rotary's offer. Of the meeting, Renouf was to later write: "It was an historic moment, with representatives of the Ministry of Health, Rotary, WHO, and UNICEF present, for we were not only committing ourselves to the expenditure of substantial Rotary funds on a project the like of which we had never previously undertaken — in our alliance with agencies of the United Nations we were putting Rotary's reputation on the line for all to see."

Renouf received further encouragement for the Philippines experiment from District Governor John Sever, who was then chief of the Infectious Diseases branch of the U.S. National Institutes of Health and had worked with OPV-developer Sabin. "If a single vaccine were to be selected for the 3-H program, I would recommend poliomyelitis," Dr. Sever wrote in May 1979 in response to Renouf's inquiry.

The RI Board gave the green light to the Philippines 3-H project later that month. PolioPlus had taken root.

Overleaf: Dr. Otto Austel and other Rotarians in the medical professions have volunteered their time and skills in polio-endemic and at-risk countries.

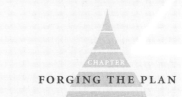

FORGING THE PLAN

FORGING THE PLAN

WITH APPROVAL OF the Philippines polio immunization project in 1979, PolioPlus entered a six-year period in which Rotary explored and tested its capacity to help deliver vaccines to children.

Two developments during this time proved critical to the life of the 3-H program and may in fact have prevented its early death. First, Renouf's successors as president strongly supported 3-H and its polio immunization component. Second, the 1980 Council on Legislation adopted a resolution directing the RI Board of Directors and the Trustees of The Rotary Foundation to continue working together to develop 3-H projects. Moreover, the resolution authorized the expenditure of Rotary Foundation funds on 3-H projects, in addition to the $7.2 million raised for the 75th Anniversary Fund.

This clear mandate from Rotary's highest legislative body helped to rebuff repeated attempts to kill the 3-H program in its infancy. "We may have been led to go too far too fast," said a leading critic of the program. Rotary

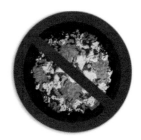

Distributed by the thousands, this "Stop Polio" button depicting the poliovirus became the symbol of Rotary's program to eradicate polio.

Opposite: A historic moment: On 29 September 1979, RI President James Bomar gave two drops of oral polio vaccine to a young girl in Manila, thus launching a 25-year effort that so far has protected some two billion children against polio.

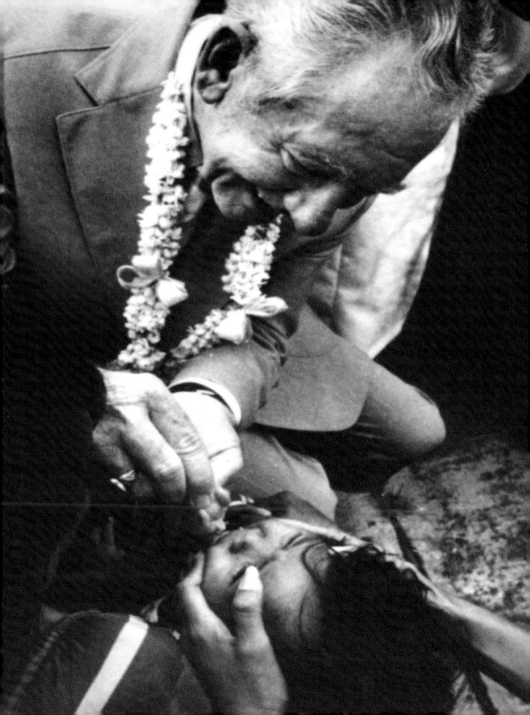

policies proscribing corporate action by Rotary International were immutable in his view and those of a few past RI presidents. "I would much prefer," he said, "to have the cynics accuse Rotary of not doing anything because it does not attempt by corporate action to solve world-encircling economic and social ills, than to see Rotary impair its effectiveness in areas in which it has achieved over a long period of years successful and widespread results through encouraging the individual to act." He attacked the 3-H concept itself by quoting Nobel laureate Linus Pauling: "The goal of the human race should not be to have as many people on earth as can possibly be kept alive . . . but rather to have only that number of people who can lead good lives." Such sentiments were not in tune with the vision of Rotarians worldwide. They were ready to take on a major world problem.

The Philippine agreement was signed on 29 September 1979 by RI President James L. Bomar. After the signing, Bomar and other Rotarians went to a Manila schoolyard, where 100 children, many of whom were crippled, had gathered with their parents to receive the vaccine. The location of the event symbolized Rotary's commitment to provide vaccine for six million children and a pledge by Philippine Rotarians to promote immunization through education programs. Bomar lifted an infant girl from her mother's arms and placed two drops of oral polio vaccine on her tongue. As he did so, a young boy, paralyzed from the waist down, tugged on Bomar's trousers, turned his smiling face upward, and said: "Thank you, Rotary. She's my sister." With those two drops, Rotary embarked on a path that would eventually reach more than two billion children.

Fear of polio's crippling effects spurred parents to bring increasing numbers of children to their nation's health centers. There, the children

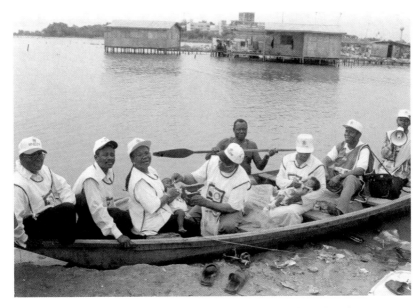

National Immunization Days target every child under the age of five. Rotarian volunteers employ nearly every kind of transportation to reach all communities, such as this village on a river in Nigeria.

received the polio vaccine and often were vaccinated against other communicable diseases. By July 1980, polio vaccine was reaching 90 percent of children ages five and under, the target age group. By 1982, the number of polio cases in the Philippines had decreased by 68 percent. With the Philippines 3-H immunization project as a model, similar projects were launched in Cambodia, Haiti, Morocco, Paraguay, and Sierra Leone. These were to further shape Rotary's approach to immunizing children.

In 1981-82, RI President Stanley E. McCaffrey appointed a committee to solicit suggestions for "new ideas and constructive innovations designed to accomplish our objectives of service to humanity." The New Horizons Committee received nearly 3,000 ideas from Rotarians worldwide, including a specific proposal from John Sever that Rotary should "support the goals of immunization for children and the eradication of polio by the year 2005."

Although polio immunization already had been demonstrated as a 3-H project, Sever's proposal offered a specific target. The committee endorsed the proposal and sent it to the Board of Directors, which agreed to the goal of "immunizing all the world's children against polio by the time of the 100th anniversary of Rotary International in the year 2005." The decision represented a quantum leap in commitment. "If we had realized all the complexity, that decision would never have been made," New Horizons Committee Chair Cliff Dochterman later said.

A major aspect of that complexity centered on a global debate about the best strategy for immunizing children in developing countries. At a 1982 meeting of the 3-H Committee, incoming RI President Carlos Canseco, an allergist with extensive public health experience in Mexico, stated that there was no hope of eradicating polio with the sporadic projects then being funded by 3-H grants. Eradication, he said, would require annual, mass immunization campaigns in *all* polio-endemic countries, campaigns that would flood the under-five population with vaccine virus and capture the benefits of passive, or secondary, immunization. If sustained for a number of years, reaching at least 80 percent of the target population, polio could disappear. Given the weak health-system infrastructures in many polio-endemic countries, routine immunization programs could not and were not reaching sufficient

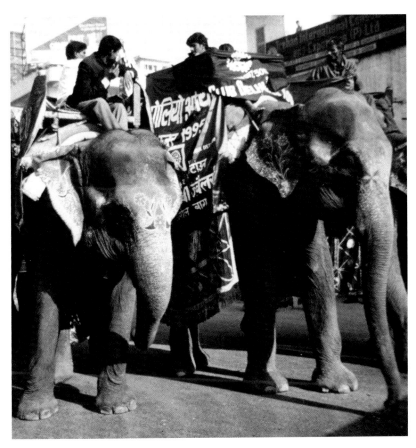

Intensive publicity efforts help spread the word about the value of immunization. Polio immunization days have provided millions of children their first contacts with public health systems.
Photo by Hugh Horan

numbers of children. In the early 1970s, for example, only 1 in 20 newborns in developing countries was immunized against communicable diseases.

WHO's Expanded Programme on Immunization, however, opposed mass immunizations targeting only one disease. The EPI had been launched at the 1978 International Conference on Primary Health Care, in Alma-Ata, USSR (now Kazakhstan), with the goal of reaching 90 percent of newborns with a protective course of vaccines against polio, measles, tuberculosis, diphtheria, pertussis (whooping cough), and tetanus.

The EPI was being carried out as a core program of a steadily expanding and sustainable system of primary health care. Despite the success of the smallpox eradication program and its "vertical" approach of targeting a single disease, WHO believed money and resources were better spent on broad-front, "horizontal" efforts that allowed countries to focus on those diseases that represented the highest rates of morbidity and mortality.

Rotary's intention to concentrate on polio, just one of the six diseases targeted by EPI, sharpened the vertical versus horizontal debate. The merits of the competing strategies were argued in meetings among health professionals, development agencies, donors, and others, producing so many reports "that we could have solved the world hunger problems had we printed them all on rice paper," one public health professional wryly observed.

Without expertise in public health affairs, and uncomfortable with choosing between competing viewpoints among global health professionals, Rotary set out to find a compromise strategy faithful to its own dream of polio eradication yet supportive of broader immunization goals.

That strategy began to take shape early in Canseco's year as RI president in 1984-85. He appointed Sever to head the 11-member Polio 2005 Committee and invited Sabin to serve as special consultant. It met in early July 1984. Having witnessed the dramatic results of mass campaigns in the Soviet Union, Brazil, Cuba, and elsewhere, Sabin saw in Rotary an angel with the answer to his dream of a polio-free world: a million men of influence in more than 100 countries who could marshal the money and manpower to deliver oral polio vaccine to children, house to house, in twice-yearly campaigns. He proposed the formation of a global polio immunization task force that would help each polio-endemic nation plan and mobilize the logistics of such massive campaigns. Sabin, a heroic figure and household name in many countries, was a convincing advocate. But how much would such a program cost, and how would it work?

The committee asked RI General Secretary Herbert Pigman, who had headed Rotary's program development for 13 years, to explore such a program. He conferred with James Grant, executive director of UNICEF, the United Nations agency that coordinates vaccine procurement and delivery on behalf of many donor nation development agencies and is a leader in training programs for social mobilization. Together, they explored a three-part

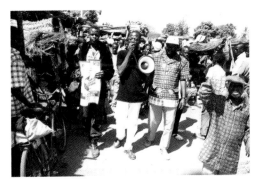

"Polio immunization day!" Aiming for 100 percent coverage, volunteers equipped with portable speakers reach villages not served by radio or television.

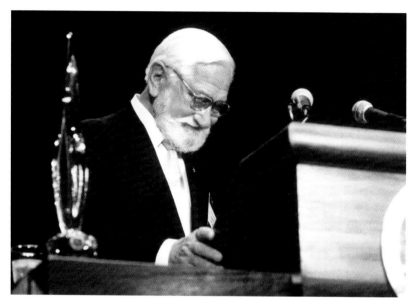

Dr. Albert Sabin's dramatic plea at the 1985 RI Convention fired Rotarians' resolve to accelerate plans for a $120 million fundraising campaign for polio vaccine. "Unless there are changes made," Sabin warned, "when Rotary is 100 years old, there will be eight million more paralyzed children."

role for Rotary that would complement the work of UNICEF, WHO, and other major players: provide massive amounts of oral polio vaccine for five years, help develop political support, and mobilize at the community level to conduct public-awareness campaigns on the value of parents immunizing their children. Grant, Pigman, and Sever estimated that the cost of providing oral polio vaccine to polio-endemic countries would be $120 million, based on a formula of six doses at $0.04 per dose for each of 100 million newborns for five years.

In October 1984, Pigman presented to the Polio 2005 Committee a two-page memorandum incorporating Sabin's ideas for an expert task force, a goal of $120 million for vaccine purchase, and a plan that Rotarians in polio-endemic countries would team up with their ministries of health to mobilize volunteer support for mass immunization drives. Endorsed by the committee and adopted by the RI Board and Foundation Trustees, the program was later to acquire a new name: PolioPlus. The word *polio* signaled Rotary's vertical attack on the poliovirus; *plus* referred to Rotary's horizontal bonus of assistance in the areas of managerial experience, political will, funding, and community organization, all of which would help national health systems boost immunization levels of their children against polio as well as the five other diseases targeted by EPI.

Many Rotarians assumed that $120 million in vaccine would eradicate the disease. In fact, PolioPlus was designed to provide vaccine for only five years, a period deemed sufficient to help nations put the virus on the road to elimination. The true dimensions of the challenge — and its price tag of more than $3 billion — would not become known for several years.

With Rotary's adoption of a basic plan for its participation in the global drive to immunize children, the pace of polio eradication began to quicken. On 14 May 1985, the Pan American Health Organization (PAHO), a regional arm of WHO, announced its plan to eradicate polio from the Americas by 1990. Canseco led a successful effort to obtain formal recognition for Rotary as a consultant agency to WHO, overcoming the skepticism of WHO Director-General Halfdan Mahler, who considered Rotary, with no track record in public health, just another do-good organization whose support would fade after it had grabbed a few headlines.

Thus the stage was set for RI President Canseco's announcement of the details of PolioPlus to thousands of enthusiastic Rotarians at the RI Convention in Kansas City, Kansas, USA. Sabin, present to receive the Rotary Award for World Understanding, challenged the audience. "Unless there are changes made," he said, "20 years from now, when Rotary is 100 years old, there will be an accumulated eight million more paralyzed children in the world . . . probably 800,000 deaths."

Rotary revealed PolioPlus to world leaders in October 1985 at a conference of heads of state assembled in New York for the 40th anniversary of the United Nations. The occasion was a UNICEF-sponsored gathering announcing a universal childhood-immunization program and its goal to raise immunization levels worldwide to 80 percent by 1990. It would require a massive effort. In his remarks, Grant foresaw the role that nongovernmental organizations would play. "It is upon them," he said, "that we shall depend for the ultimate success of our venture."

Rotary was asked to speak on behalf of 600 nongovernmental organization leaders represented at the meeting. Pigman unveiled Rotary's plan to join the battle against childhood infectious diseases by specifically targeting polio. The $120 million pledge by a private sector organization, backed by a volunteer army of one million community leaders, was unprecedented in public health history. It electrified the meeting. "It was a proud moment for Rotary," Pigman said later. "It was also an audacious moment. We didn't have a dime in the bank to back up that pledge."

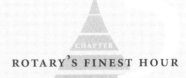

ROTARY'S FINEST HOUR

ROTARY'S FINEST HOUR

IN 1984-85, ROTARY'S membership was approaching one million. Raising $120 million dollars from such a large group of successful business and professional leaders seemed a readily attainable goal, especially if the appeal were to be stretched out over 20 years to reduce risk to ongoing financial support of The Rotary Foundation.

Rotarians were increasing their support of the Foundation and its expanding menu of programs. In the five-year period beginning with Rotary year 1979-80, they had contributed an average of $16,175,119 a year to the Foundation's Annual Programs Fund. An additional $5 million to $6 million a year for PolioPlus, it was reasoned, would not unduly jeopardize this level of support, especially if Rotarians invited the general public to contribute.

The strategy for a 20-year appeal was soon scuttled for several reasons. Sabin's impassioned plea to the Kansas City convention, warning of eight million more paralyzed children in the next two decades, escalated Rotarians' resolve to act promptly. In a mobile society where the poliovirus could quickly reinfect polio-free nations, the epidemiology of polio militated against a piecemeal approach to eradication. And experienced fundraisers counseled that a lengthy campaign probably could not be sustained. Rotary's leaders, gauging the sentiments expressed at the Kansas City convention, decided to take a gamble. They compressed the fundraising timetable to three years. Furthermore, Rotarians themselves would be expected to contribute a substantial part of the $120 million.

The first year of the three-year fundraising campaign, 1985-86, was devoted to educating Rotarians about the polio program, planning the logistics of the fundraising campaign, and identifying and training campaign leaders.

The RI Board appointed the seven-member International PolioPlus Committee to coordinate the campaign, chaired by Past RI Director Les Wright. The campaign structure consisted of an executive director and staff, 11 international coordinators, 84 national coordinators, 44 national or multinational PolioPlus committees, and 3,300 area coordinators — a cadre of 3,900 volunteers, all of whom needed tools and training to enable them to carry their message to Rotarians in 23,000 communities in 161 countries. Wright, a university president, realized the need for professional counsel for such a massive and complex undertaking. New York-based Community Counseling Services (CCS) was selected. Of the nine firms interviewed, CCS best appreciated the potential for grassroots support and the effective use of Rotary volunteers. CCS staff came on board in May 1986.

Even before the campaign had formally started, Rotarians began to raise funds, and some had set goals. Individuals sent contributions. By the end of the year, $227,000 had been raised. "It was like trying to build an airplane while we were already in the air," said one CCS staffer.

The overall responsibility of training, motivating, and coordinating the efforts of this massive volunteer structure fell on the shoulders of Past District Governor Walter Maddocks, a Bermuda barrister turned Kentucky horse farmer whose service as vice chair of the 1986 Council on Legislation had put the spotlight on his leadership abilities. Maddocks accepted the call and served as a volunteer for two years, earning the plaudits of all Rotarians and recognition from the U.S. government as one of 18 outstanding volunteers.

With Maddocks at the throttle and ably supported by the full-time volunteer service of Rotarian Jack Blane, RI staff, and CCS, the wheels of the massive campaign structure began to turn. Ten clubs were selected as models to test rank-and-file response to a carefully orchestrated appeal. Each club was assigned a share of the $120 million goal. Together, contributions from the 10 clubs tripled the total amount of their shares. Clearly, the quest for a polio-free world resonated well with Rotarians.

The "share" concept, however, was not without criticism. The formula for a club's PolioPlus share was based on its previous contributions to The Rotary Foundation. The premise, that most gifts will come from those who have already given, was standard in North American philanthropic endeavors, but some clubs that had given generously to The Rotary Foundation complained of being unfairly burdened. Some clubs that had previously provided little or no support to the Foundation complained that their share was so low as to be insulting. Some national PolioPlus fundraising committees, protesting that the campaign's fundraising tools and techniques were foreign to their cultures, devised their own goals and procedures. Although the global goal was $120 million, planners anticipated that some clubs would not participate in PolioPlus. They compensated for this by devising a share formula that would achieve a goal substantially in excess of the $120 million target.

The campaign progressed well. The creativity and zeal of Rotarians in raising PolioPlus funds astounded the CCS professional staff. In addition to their personal contributions, which included several large gifts, such as a $1 million contribution from Chicago Rotarian Clement Stone, Rotarians conducted hundreds of fundraising activities: raffles, wine-tasting parties, golf tournaments, chicken-plucking contests, carnivals, and car rallies. In France, a street appeal collected $3 million. Verneil Martin, wife of a past district governor, gathered recipes and published a cookbook that raised $1 million. A Dutch Rotaract club built and pedaled an amphibious craft powered by 36 bicycles across the English Channel and through three European countries, garnering $210,000 for PolioPlus and enormous publicity for the campaign. A benefit concert by violinist Itzhak Perlman, a polio survivor, raised $140,000. Celebrities including entertainers Helen Hayes and Bob Hope, baseball player Mark McGwire, and photographer Lord Snowdon lent support. Appeals to governments brought a total of $9,929,000, including a $6 million grant from USAID, $1.3 million from Belgium, $1 million from the Canadian Public Health Association, and £1 million (roughly US$1.47 million at the time) from the British Ministry of Overseas Development. Corporate contributions came from Baxter Healthcare, BellSouth, Coca-Cola, Connaught Labs, DeBeers, Hershey, and Lederle Laboratories.

By September 1987, $50 million had been contributed; by January 1988, the total hit $100 million. Money and pledges were rolling in at a rate of $1 million a day. Fifteen bookkeepers scrambled to acknowledge contributions, calculate currency exchange rates, and record, report, and deposit the money. On 3 February 1988, the total reached $120 million. Maddocks thereafter embargoed news of the global total, reserving the final result for announcement at the RI Convention, just three months away.

Philadelphia, known as the City of Brotherly Love, was an auspicious host city for the 1988 RI Convention. The convention stage and hall were carefully prepared for the announcement of the campaign results. Maddocks telephoned his staff the night before to get a final update: More than $2 million in cash and pledges had come in that very day.

On 24 May in the convention hall, RI President Charles Keller called Wright and Maddocks to the podium. Then Maddocks asked the chair of each of the 44 multinational or national fundraising committees to announce his committee's results. As the cumulative totals appeared on a large screen, additional "victory lights" ringing the auditorium flashed on. Suspense mounted as the report of the 43rd committee inched the total just above $100 million. Then Herb Brown, U.S. committee chair and last to report, announced the U.S. total: $119 million. "We did it!" Maddocks shouted. "We're over the goal — $219,350,499!" Fifteen thousand balloons cascaded from the ceiling. A band marched down the aisles among thousands of people who were applauding, crying, and hugging one another. Seldom had the City of Brotherly Love witnessed such a joyous, emotion-filled scene.

Further good news came with the announcement that 12 days earlier the World Health Assembly had unanimously adopted a resolution to eradicate polio. WHO Director-General Mahler introduced the resolution himself, saying, "If it can be done, it must be done." In a message to the Philadelphia convention, Mahler praised Rotary. "As business and professional leaders, you have helped to change attitudes toward immunization," he said. A videotape of the Philadelphia celebration would later bear the title "Rotary's Finest Hour."

The PolioPlus campaign total rose to $247 million by the end of the Rotary year. The campaign's success stunned the Rotary world as well as Rotary's partners in the field of public health. Eighty-five percent of Rotary's 23,000 clubs had responded, reporting gifts that averaged $6,248. More than

Opposite: Rotary clubs worldwide drew community support to their campaign to raise funds to combat polio. Individual contributions ranged from a few yen to a gift of $1 million.

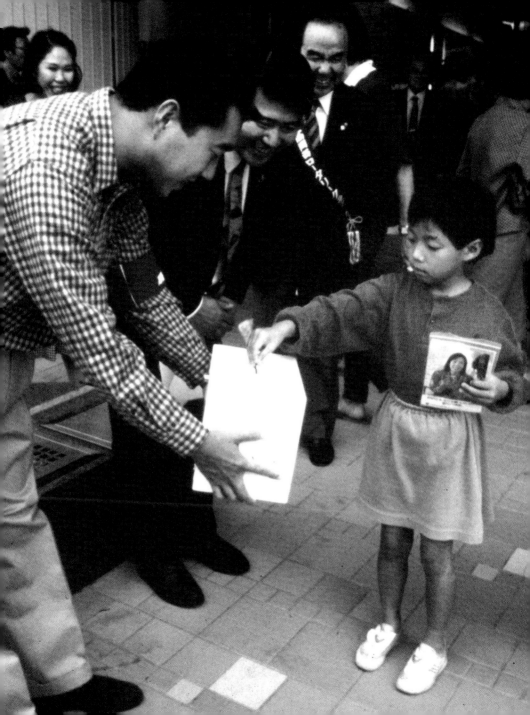

200 Rotarians had made major gifts of $25,000 or more. Rotary had not only met but doubled the commitment made to world leaders in October 1985.

It was a time for celebration, indeed. But it was not the last time that the world would look to Rotary to fuel the engines of the global polio eradication program.

Victory balloons cascade at the 1988 RI Convention in Philadelphia with the stunning announcement that Rotarians had surpassed the PolioPlus fundraising goal by $100 million. The campaign total eventually climbed to $247 million.

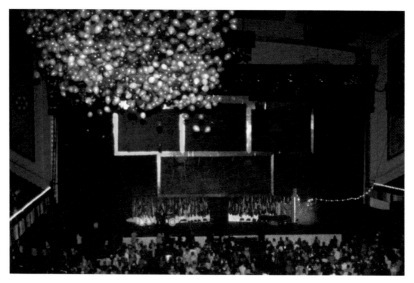

AMERICAS, THE PROVING GROUND

AMERICAS, THE PROVING GROUND

CONCURRENT WITH ITS effort to raise $120 million for the purchase of polio vaccine, Rotary launched work on the second part of its PolioPlus commitment: marshaling Rotary manpower and resources in polio-endemic countries to help deliver that vaccine to children. The PAHO, the WHO region serving the Americas, would be the proving ground for a polio eradication strategy destined to be adopted worldwide. It was also the region in which Rotarians developed and refined their role: funding, social mobilization, application of business know-how to obstacles to vaccine distribution, promotion of cooperation among external aid partners, and political advocacy. Guiding Rotary's role in this strategy was the responsibility of the Rotary Immunization Task Force.

In 1986, Rotary leaders interviewed several public health professionals for the job of task force director. They soon concluded that mobilizing Rotary's army of volunteers required someone with a thorough knowledge of the organization's structure, culture, and administrative machinery. They asked Herb Pigman, who was retiring as RI general secretary on 30 June 1986, to head the task force, choose its members, and guide its work. The day after his retirement, Pigman packed his bags for an assignment that was to include more than 60 country visits in Asia, Africa, and Latin America during the next 36 months.

The technical expert leading the PAHO attack on polio was Dr. Ciro de Quadros, a Brazilian epidemiologist and veteran of the smallpox eradication program. De Quadros was convinced that with the necessary sufficient political and social will, polio could be eradicated in the entire region, which had already seen successes; polio had been eliminated in Cuba in 1962, and Brazil's National Immunization

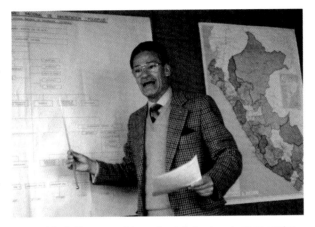

National PolioPlus committees direct Rotary's volunteer armies in polio-endemic countries. Gustavo Gross (above) organized Rotary's input of 28,000 lunches, 840 vehicles, and other logistical support for Peru's first National Immunization Day.

Days, inspired by Sabin's help in 1980, had reached 20 million children and reduced polio cases from an average of 100 to 200 a month to fewer than 20. But there were formidable problems: disease surveillance was marginal or nonexistent in many PAHO countries. Few laboratories could support case investigation. Guerrilla warfare disrupted some countries. An estimated $90 million was needed in international donor support.

But the promise of Rotary's PolioPlus program, with its initial commitment of $10 million in funding for PAHO countries, had helped to tip the scales. Rotarians had demonstrated their effectiveness in social mobilization in Paraguay and other countries. On 14 May 1985, PAHO

Director Carlyle Guerra de Macedo, flanked by RI President Carlos Canseco and other partners, announced that PAHO would seek to eradicate polio from the Western Hemisphere by 1990. At that time, there were 1,000 reported cases of polio in 11 countries in the region.

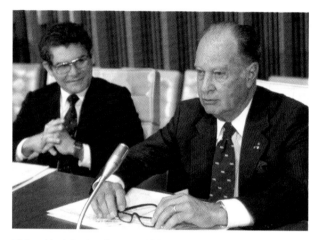

RI President Carlos Canseco (right) pledged Rotary's full support of PAHO's historic 1985 decision to eradicate polio in the Western Hemisphere.

With PolioPlus contributions flowing in, the pace of Rotary's work quickened. At RI World Headquarters, John Stucky and his associate Michael McQuestion managed the grant process. Stucky had joined the staff in 1979 following a career as missionary in Brazil and with the Medical Assistance Program, an organization that distributes donated vaccines and medical supplies to needy countries, and both he and McQuestion approached their tasks with missionary zeal.

Typical PolioPlus grants provided a five-year supply of oral polio vaccine. The vaccine was purchased through UNICEF, which had negotiated with vaccine manufacturers a global, three-tiered pricing system that provided the vaccine to poor nations for as little as $0.04 per dose. Rich nations paid the most. The cost per dose to a private physician in the United States, for example, exceeded $10. Middle-income nations paid less. Each grant also included a modest amount for the work of national PolioPlus committees. This seed money proved catalytic. A study conducted in one country revealed that each PolioPlus dollar invested in Rotary support activities generated more than $2 worth of locally donated materiel or services.

On National Immunization Days (NIDs), Rotarians, spouses, family members, friends, and often employees turned out to immunize children at immunization posts and in follow-up house-to-house visits. In Lima, Peru, for example, National PolioPlus Committee Chair Gustavo Gross established a "war room" in which large maps showed Lima barrios to which Rotarians and other volunteers were assigned. On the appointed day, polio vaccine, which needs refrigeration, was carried in ice-filled Styrofoam containers from central stores to immunization sites. Lima alone required 10 tons of ice for its immunization day. Rotarians prepared 28,000 lunches for health workers and volunteers, deployed 840 vehicles to transport supplies, and assisted at 2,300 vaccination posts.

Immunization days, some of which required negotiation with guerrilla forces to guarantee safety for health workers and volunteers, caused polio cases to plummet. The success of the PAHO strategy for eradicating polio, however, hinged on improved surveillance, or nationwide systems for identifying polio cases. Uniform case definitions had to be developed. Gradually, health professionals forged a four-part strategy:

1. Maintain the highest possible level of routine immunization.

2. Supplement routine immunization with mass vaccination days.

3. Conduct surveillance.

4. Use the surveillance data to identify pockets where the poliovirus
   continues to circulate and attack with mop-up immunization efforts,
   including house-to-house visits.

Acceptable standards of surveillance required that any case of acute
paralytic illness in a child under age 15 be investigated within 48 hours by
a trained epidemiologist. Two stool specimens, collected 24 hours apart,
were to be sent to a laboratory qualified to differentiate the poliovirus from
other pathogens that can cause paralysis. Eventually, a reporting network
established throughout Latin America required some 20,000 health facilities
to report weekly on any case of acute flaccid paralysis, or the absence of any.
Some Rotarians helped this process by lending use of their telephones and
fax machines. In Brazil, National PolioPlus Committee Chair Archimedes
Theodoro raised public awareness of the polio effort by publishing a book
about PolioPlus and, in the process, enlisting thousands of his fellow
pediatricians in the search for polio cases.

By 1989, only six PAHO countries reported cases. By 1990, only 18
cases were reported in the entire region, and in the next year, just 9 cases.
The last confirmed case of polio due to the wild poliovirus was detected
on 23 August 1991, in a two-year-old Peruvian boy named Luis Fermín
Tenorio. Peruvian Rotarians later cared for Luis, providing for his
rehabilitation and education.

PAHO conducted an intensive search for cases over the next three years,
offering a reward of $100 — later increased to $1,000 — to anyone reporting
an AFP case that turned out to be polio. No new cases were found.

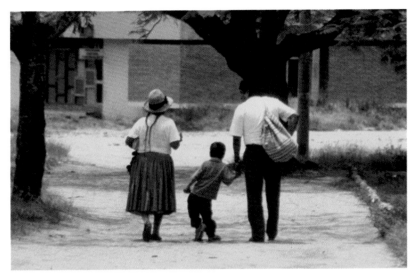

In 1994, an international commission certified the PAHO region polio-free. The last case of polio was Luis Fermín Tenorio (above) of Peru. Immunization and surveillance strategies pioneered in PAHO came to guide polio eradication efforts worldwide.

To certify that polio had indeed been eradicated in its region, PAHO created an independent International Certification Commission on Poliomyelitis Eradication, chaired by Nobel laureate Frederick C. Robbins. It established the following certification criteria (later used by other WHO regions): surveillance of acute flaccid paralysis and wild poliovirus, active search for AFP cases, and mop-up operations in high-risk areas. Tough surveillance standards were set. At least 80 percent of all health units had to report weekly the absence or presence of AFP. The system had to find at least one AFP case per 100,000 children under age 15 (not all AFP cases are caused by the poliovirus, thus the absence of any reported AFP cases could indicate a system failure). At least 80 percent of all reported paralysis cases needed to have two stool specimens processed for virus culture by a WHO-accredited laboratory within two weeks of onset of paralysis and stool investigation done for family contacts.

In September 1994, Robbins declared before an audience of Latin American health ministers gathered in Washington, D.C., that polio had been eradicated in the PAHO region. The historic moment was a proud one for PAHO, Rotary, and other organizations.

The campaign had left an impressive legacy: validation of the role of volunteer groups in public health; a cadre of trained epidemiologists; a network of virology laboratories; interagency coordinating committees; a boost in morale for public health workers; a surveillance system that could help combat other communicable diseases, such as measles; greater political awareness; and national budgets that provided increased funds for immunization.

The PAHO campaign had cost about $540 million, 80 percent of it covered by the countries themselves and the rest by donors, including $38,517,388 from Rotary International. That 80-20 ratio was to change substantially as the polio battlefield moved to economically less-developed countries in Asia and Africa.

CHAPTER 7

"SIX THOUSAND CHILDREN EVERY SECOND"

"SIX THOUSAND CHILDREN EVERY SECOND"

A S T H E F I R S T rays of the January sun touched the peaks of the
Himalayas and spread westward across the Indian subcontinent, the vast
army of three million people began to stir. In sprawling, crowded cities and in
500,000 rural villages from Kashmir to Kerala and from Assam to Rajasthan,
the banners unfurled. National Immunization Day was at hand. India, a
nation of more than one billion people, once again was mobilizing to deliver
a knockout blow to an old and feared nemesis: polio. By nightfall that Sunday,
and in the two days of house-to-house visits that followed, the army of health
workers and volunteers would achieve a feat of staggering dimensions: the
immunization of more than 150 million children against polio.

In Mumbai, capital of Maharashtra, the alarm clock rang at 0500 in the
home of Dr. Chandrasekhar Joshi. The 50-year-old surgeon, known as Chandru
by his fellow Rotarians in the Rotary Club of Bombay Queens Necklace, moved
through his 30-minute hatha yoga routine to prepare himself for the rigors of
the day ahead. As he downed a hearty breakfast of potatoes, onions, and rice
prepared by his wife, Rohini, he mentally reviewed the details of his assignment.

Joshi had drawn a particularly challenging task: supervising immunization
operations in a crowded and fetid neighborhood in the heart of Dharavi,
reputed to be Asia's largest slum and notorious as a hideout for drug dealers,
prostitutes, and gunrunners. It was also home to 100,000 children. He would
serve as a coordinator and troubleshooter, checking to ensure that each of the
250 immunization posts set up for the day was staffed by two government

health workers plus three volunteers, two of whom would be women (for households that prohibit men who aren't relatives from entering), and that oral polio vaccine was in place and properly refrigerated.

By 0630 Joshi was on his cell phone to a fellow Rotarian. "Any problems with getting the vaccine from the cold-storage center to the booths?" The report was reassuring: The Rotary Club of Mumbai Downtown had purchased and recently delivered 3,000 vaccine carriers.

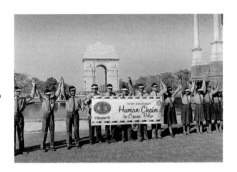

In India, National Immunization Days engage more than 350,000 volunteers from the family of Rotary, including these Rotaractors who helped publicize the event with a 550,000-person human chain.

Fifteen minutes later, Joshi was on the road, visiting booths. A friendly wave from a booth team indicated all was right. But some booths had problems. Mothers and fathers had been queuing up since 0700. Vaccines had arrived an hour late. A fight had erupted at another booth. The supply of balloons and whistles had run out, disappointing kids; parents were balking at getting their kids immunized. Frantic cell phone calls filled the void. Mobile immunization teams, he observed, were in place at bus and railway stations. Joshi made a mental note to ring up fellow Rotarian Lata Rao, who was responsible for getting candies to these mobile teams.

A dozen "miking" teams were roaming various neighborhoods in auto-rickshaws, urging people through megaphones to take their children to the

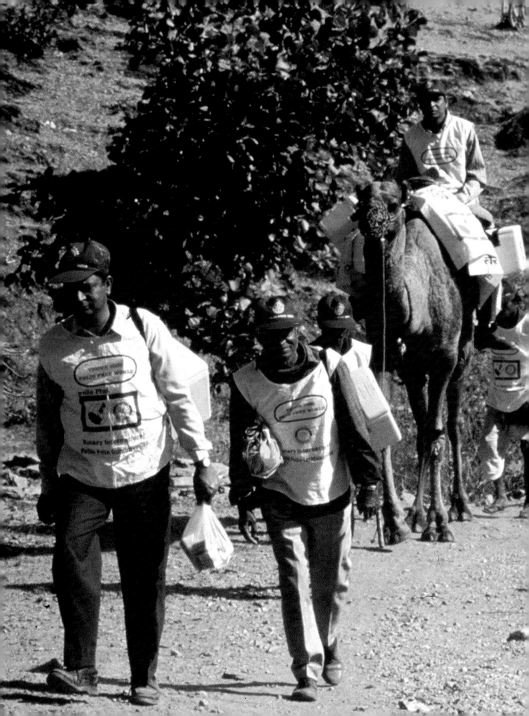

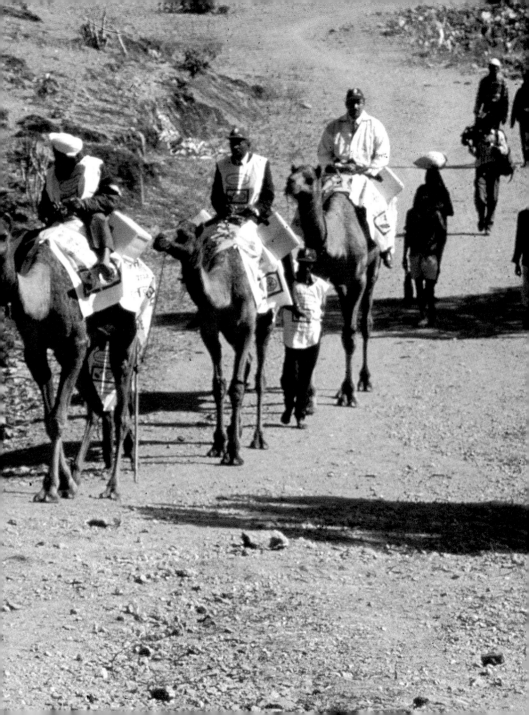

booths. A video van donated by Rotary was already attracting crowds of kids to see film clips of movie hero Amitabh Bachchan. UNICEF had enlisted him as an ambassador to deliver a message about the importance of polio immunization. Surveys had shown that 92 percent of mothers put great faith in an appeal by this Indian film superstar.

Fifty booth visits later, Joshi's hectic pace began to slow. By 1200 at Ravalwadi market, over 70 percent of the target group (children under age five) had come to the booth. Supplies of caps, sunshades, balloons, and whistles were exhausted, and so was the staff who had worked for hours under the temporary tent warmed by a hot sun, squeezing two drops of oral polio vaccine into each child's mouth, thanking parents and reassuring them when necessary. Joshi checked the insulated vaccine carrier. Good. The ice was still present. The color-sensitive temperature monitor on each 20-dose vial of oral polio vaccine showed that the vaccine was still potent. He shook hands with each of the booth staff, ordered a round of soft drinks at his expense, and headed home. For Joshi, it was a strenuous day. But he had the satisfaction that he was not alone in his nation's quest. Every member of the Rotary Club of Bombay Queens Necklace, one of 73 Rotary clubs in Mumbai, had volunteered this day, donning the distinctive yellow PolioPlus vests and reporting to their stations. And across the nation, so had 350,000 volunteers from the family of Rotary, including club members, spouses, Interactors, Rotaractors, Rotary Community Corps members, and Inner Wheel members.

Overleaf: NIDs in India require transport of oral polio vaccine to 650,000 immunization booths, employing every means of transportation, from helicopters to camels. Four months in the planning, each NID reaches some 150 million children.
Photo by Marcus Oleniuk

For Joshi and his fellow Rotarians, however, the task was not over. The following two days were spent trudging through rutted lanes muddy with raw sewage, checking shanty dwellings to find any child who had not been brought to a booth on Sunday. Each dwelling was chalked with a symbol marking the date and number of children immunized. Those who had been immunized were easily identified by indelible ink used to mark the child's finger.

National Immunization Days in India constitute the world's largest public-health events. Detailed planning begins three to four months before the NID. Approximately 650,000 immunization booths are set up in locations throughout the country, including airports, rail and bus stations, and amusement parks. Approximately 225 million doses of oral polio vaccine (cost: $24 million) are stockpiled, as are thousands of vaccine carriers and hundreds of tons of ice. House-to-house follow-up efforts require 1.3 million teams, each with two or three members. Nearly every form of communication is employed: drum beating; public announcements broadcast from rickshaws and scooters; television and radio appeals from celebrities, clerics, and political leaders; street plays; road shows; and video vans. A vast fleet of trucks, cars, boats, airplanes, helicopters, elephants, camels, donkeys, and mules is deployed. Public health leaders from other countries were astounded by India's ability to reach 150 million children in a single day. "It's simple," said one Rotary PolioPlus leader. "You just need to gear up to immunize 6,000 children every second."

The strong advocacy of Rotary leaders was critical to India's decision to undertake National Immunization Days. Such a strategy, coupled with a

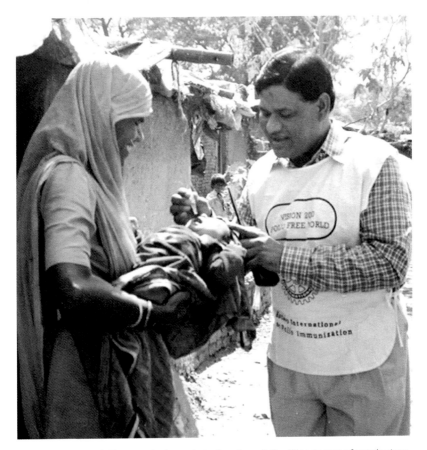

Yellow vests identify Rotary volunteers in India, where 1.3 million teams of vaccinators go house to house to ensure no child is overlooked. *Overleaf:* An indelible dye marks the fingers of children who have received the polio vaccine.
Overleaf photo by Jean-Marc Giboux

massive improvement in surveillance, was critical to global success; India was the largest reservoir of the poliovirus, experiencing each year about 70 percent of the world's reported polio cases. At the urging of Rotary and its major partners, India's first NID was held in 1995, reaching 82 million children and attracting new public and private supporters along with national and state government support. In later years, when program fatigue threatened, Rotary was the private-sector leader in keeping the flame alive. In 2002, India's National PolioPlus Committee organized Banners to Banish Polio, a competition for Rotary clubs, schools, and other groups. Each was asked to create a cloth banner measuring 2 meters (6.5 feet) to promote polio immunization. Entries poured in from the entire nation. When all were stitched together, the banners stretched for more than 31 miles, boosting public awareness and, incidentally, earning a place in *Guinness World Records*.

Rotary's leadership drew others to the cause, including young adults of India's National Social Service, the National Cadet Corps, and auxiliary nurse midwives, government-employed primary care advocates. To boost the spirit of teamwork, Rotary bought 26,000 distinctive saris for auxiliary nurse midwives in Uttar Pradesh.

Although they differ in scope, the logistics and operations of National Immunization Days bear much similarity among countries. They target children under age five, regardless of previous immunization status. Delivery of oral polio vaccine is critical. Because it can be destroyed by excessive heat, the vaccine must be kept at no more than 40 degrees Fahrenheit and rapidly transported to immunization posts from central cold stores.

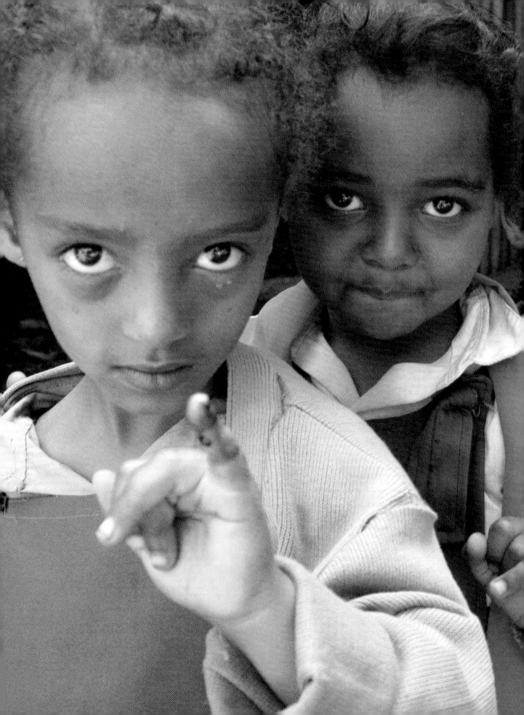

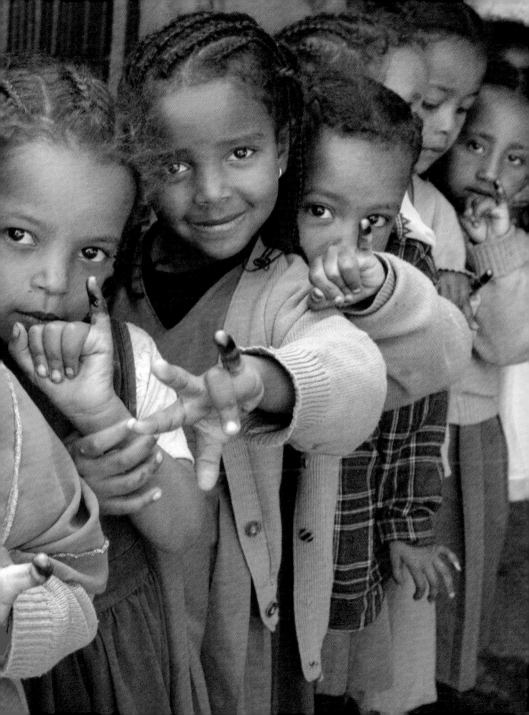

The NID strategy works. In 2002, 500 million children were vaccinated in 93 countries, using about two billion doses of vaccine. NIDs coupled with routine delivery of polio vaccine brought a precipitous decline in the number of polio cases: from 350,000 in 1985 to fewer than 1,000 in 2002. More than two billion children received oral polio vaccine, resulting in five million children or adults, mainly in the developing world, avoiding death or paralysis from polio. More than one million Rotarians have contributed to the success of these efforts through their personal services, by enlisting hundreds of thousands of other volunteers, through political advocacy, and by contributing millions of dollars of in-kind services such as vehicles, fuel, communications equipment, posters, public announcements, and other means of mobilizing public support.

Despite India's vast size and population, disparate languages, and thousands of villages, many of whose inhabitants had never read a book or traveled faster than a bullock cart, Rotary was able to play a crucial role in social mobilization. It had both the resolve and the manpower — some 100,000 members in 1,900 communities — to back it up. It was, however, a different story for other parts of Asia and for African countries in need of similar private-sector leadership for their campaigns. Rotary's membership in several such countries was relatively small, a factor that was to place extraordinary burdens on the few clubs and members who struggled to advance the goals of the PolioPlus program.

IT'S A STUPID DOG THAT BARKS AT AN ELEPHANT

IT'S A STUPID DOG THAT BARKS AT AN ELEPHANT

— African proverb

THE RAPID PROGRESS of the Global Polio Eradication Initiative was due in large part to a timely decision by the Trustees of The Rotary Foundation. Following the press conference announcing the adoption of the World Health Assembly resolution, Dr. Rafe Henderson, director of WHO's Expanded Programme on Immunization, had told Pigman, then director of the Rotary Immunization Task Force, that little would happen as the result of this resolution unless WHO could obtain funds to hire a small team of technical experts who can give the program leadership and continuity. The Foundation Trustees responded by giving WHO a core grant of $5.3 million to hire a polio campaign coordinator in Geneva and counterparts in five of WHO's six regions.

It was to be the most important grant in the life of the PolioPlus program. The polio eradication initiative, as it came to be known by WHO, its architect, soon blossomed into the largest program in the history of public health, engaging thousands of health professionals and 20 million volunteers. Spurred by a series of successes, Rotary, national overseas-aid agencies, and private-sector firms committed nearly $3 billion in donor resources to supplement the meager budgets of polio-endemic countries. The funds were used to buy vaccine, create surveillance systems, forge a global network of 146 viral laboratories, provide training, and support NIDs and other supplementary immunization activities. The number of polio-endemic countries steadily decreased.

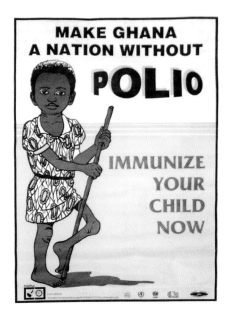

**MAKE GHANA
A NATION WITHOUT
POLIO**

**IMMUNIZE
YOUR
CHILD
NOW**

Despite economic problems and civil wars in some countries, Africa made spectacular progress in combating polio.

In an October 2000 ceremony held in Kyoto, Japan, the WHO Western Pacific region (37 countries including the world's most populous nation, the People's Republic of China) was certified polio-free. This significant accomplishment confirmed that the four-part strategy pioneered in the Americas could be successfully applied to a region of highly diverse cultures, economies, and health infrastructures.

Between 1995 and 2000, a coordinated program of NIDs in 18 high-risk countries in the WHO European and Eastern Mediterranean regions, dubbed Operation MECACAR (after the geographical regions targeted — Eastern Mediterranean, the Caucasus, and Central Asian Republics), reached 65 million children each year. It effectively stopped polio and opened the door to the certification of the European region (870 million people in 51 nations) in June 2002.

Despite these regional victories, it became clear that the global campaign would miss WHO's year 2000 target. At the close of the century, 20 countries still harbored the poliovirus. A polio-free planet, the much anticipated gift to the children of the 21st century, would have to be postponed. But for how long? Every year's delay in finding the last case of polio would add an estimated $100 million to $150 million to the price of eradication. Because of the risk of poliovirus importation, polio-free countries with weak routine-vaccination programs would require annual National Immunization Days to protect their newborns. And in several of the African countries where the virus still circulated, ethnic suspicions, emerging diseases, civil wars, and collapsing economies threatened to derail the program and raise doubts about whether eradication could ever be achieved. "It's a stupid dog that barks at an elephant," cautions an African proverb.

At the Global Polio Partners Summit in New York in September 2000, 350 representatives of donor countries, the private sector, and polio-endemic countries met to renew their global commitment. United Nations Secretary-General Kofi Annan launched the pep rally by starting a 2005 polio countdown clock in the lobby of the UN headquarters in New York. "Our race to reach the last child is a race against time," Annan warned. "If we do not seize the chance now, the virus will regain its grip and the opportunity will elude us forever." The soft-spoken world leader, born in Ghana, knew firsthand the worsening problems in the vast continent of Africa.

Over the next three years, efforts were redoubled in the remaining polio-endemic countries, bringing victories against seemingly impossible odds. For instance, in the Democratic Republic of the Congo (formerly Zaire), a nation the size of Western Europe, 55 million people had suffered a decade of intense civil war that had caused three million deaths. In the midst of political and economic chaos, health services were totally disrupted. Despite these obstacles, a devoted band of local health workers, with help from WHO, UNICEF, Rotary,

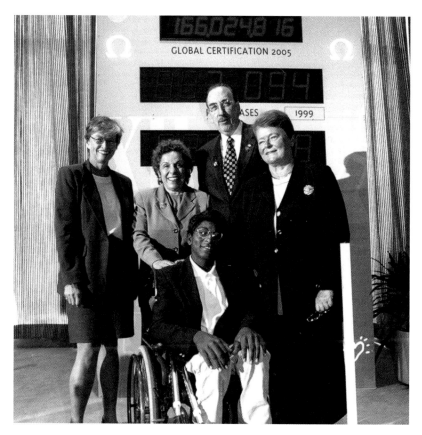

During the 2000 Global Polio Partners Summit, a case countdown clock is unveiled at UN headquarters. Among the 350 leaders attending are UNICEF Executive Director Carol Bellamy, U.S. Health and Human Services Secretary Donna Shalala, RI President Frank Devlyn, and WHO Director-General Gro Harlem Brundtland. Joining them is polio survivor Thaddeus Farrow, son of actress Mia Farrow.

and other agencies, conducted immunization days, improved surveillance, and confirmed the country's last case of polio on 29 December 2000.

In April 2003, the Global Technical Consultative Group for Poliomyelitis Eradication (TCG) adopted a major tactical shift. Concerned that donors could not continue to support costly NIDs or other supplementary immunization activities in a large number of poor nations, the TCG recommended concentrating resources on seven polio-endemic countries (Afghanistan, Egypt, India, Niger, Nigeria, Pakistan, and Somalia) plus six polio-free countries considered at highest risk of polio reinfection (Angola, Bangladesh, Democratic Republic of the Congo, Ethiopia, Nepal, and Sudan). It was a calculated risk designed to deliver a knockout blow, and it increased the need for stepping up routine immunization and surveillance in all polio-free nations. Failure to do this could quickly result in cohorts of nonimmunized newborns, fertile ground for an imported

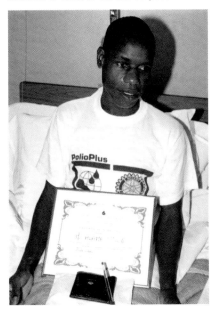

Paralyzed in the collapse of an immunization booth in Côte d'Ivoire, health worker M. Alama Silve received a commendation and a monetary award with the help of PolioPlus funds. At least 36 health workers have been disabled or killed in the war on polio.

poliovirus to touch off polio epidemics. WHO issued guidelines for managing such importations, calling for rapid investigation and confirmation of any suspected case, increased surveillance, and appropriate containment efforts such as large-scale, house-to-house mop-up operations.

In May 2003, Dr. Jong-wook Lee, a 20-year veteran of WHO, a strong advocate of polio eradication, and a good friend of Rotary's PolioPlus program leadership, succeeded Dr. Gro Harlem Brundtland as WHO director-general. He had headed the polio eradication program for the WHO Western Pacific region and later the WHO Global Programme for Vaccines and Immunizations. "I pledge to complete the eradication of polio during my tenure as director-general," Lee said during his acceptance speech at the 56th World Health Assembly.

As 2003 came to an end, fewer than 1,000 cases of polio were reported worldwide. Although Somalia had been declared polio-free, the virus stubbornly persisted in parts of the six remaining polio-endemic countries. In light of the new strategy of concentrating resources, however, a rash of poliovirus exports from infected regions to polio-free regions caused serious concern. New polio cases in Benin, Burkina Faso, Chad, Cameroun, Central African Republic, Côte d'Ivoire, Ghana, and Togo were traced to a virus strain originating in Nigeria.

In several states of northern Nigeria, Africa's most populous country, immunization efforts had collapsed. Rumors had circulated in some communities that the oral polio vaccine was contaminated with HIV or oral contraceptives. Nigeria had canceled fall 2003 immunization days and sought to allay fears by having two laboratories in South Africa confirm the absence of such contaminants. In India, similar resistance to vaccination had developed in Bihar and Uttar Pradesh, resulting in polio reinfecting several other Indian states.

The poliovirus invasion of previously polio-free areas set off alarm bells at WHO headquarters: The polio initiative was in danger of stalling. In January 2004, 13 months before Rotary was to celebrate its 100th anniversary and, hopefully, fulfillment of its dream of a polio-free world, representatives from Rotary and other major partners were called to an emergency meeting in Geneva.

In an effort to keep the initiative moving forward, health ministers or other representatives of the six polio-endemic countries renewed their nations' commitment to polio eradication, approved plans to conduct multiple campaigns to reach 250 million children, and vowed to find the last case by the end of 2004. Jointly signing the formal declaration were representatives of the four major, or spearheading, partners, including Rotary Foundation Trustee Chair James Lacy.

"The declaration is incredibly important," said Dr. Bruce Aylward, the Canadian-born pediatrician who coordinates the Global Polio Eradication Initiative. "There is a renewed commitment. Polio eradication is no longer a health issue; it is a political issue."

Indeed it was. The world had the tools to reach the goal: an effective vaccine, a proven strategy, good surveillance, money, and manpower. How effectively leaders of polio-endemic countries would prioritize and deploy their national resources would spell success or failure.

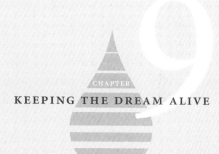

CHAPTER 9

KEEPING THE DREAM ALIVE

KEEPING THE DREAM ALIVE

Polioplus, the single largest program in Rotary's 100-year history, benefited from the talents of hundreds of Rotarians who, for more than two decades, stepped forward to provide the leadership needed to keep alive the dream of a polio-free world. They raised funds, mobilized communities, generated political support, forged partnerships, and reinforced Rotary's resolve to carry on despite problems of funding shortfalls and program fatigue. Of equal importance was their effective management of operational and financial affairs. Rotarians had committed more than $600 million from their own pockets, and millions more in volunteer and in-kind services, confident that their fellow Rotarians would provide competent stewardship of their investment.

Field operations got underway in July 1986 with the formation of the Rotary Immunization Task Force. It had four objectives:
- Offer polio-endemic countries a five-year supply of polio vaccine.
- Promote Sabin-style mass polio-immunization drives.
- Motivate Rotarians to help overcome logistical and political obstacles to polio immunization.
- Nurture partnerships with WHO, UNICEF, and other agencies at national, regional, and global levels.

Rotary had expected public health officials to greet PolioPlus with open arms. Pigman and his task force members soon discovered otherwise. Health officials were wary of Rotary, an organization with no significant experience in public health affairs, advising them on strategy and pledging to help overcome the logistical, training, and social mobilization problems that had nagged them for years. The WHO director-general himself had thrown a wet blanket on Rotary's ambitions at the World Health Assembly just two years earlier.

Rotary's financial pledge to buy oral polio vaccine, however, was too good to ignore. National-level WHO and UNICEF representatives supported local Rotarians and task force members in their negotiations. Health ministers universally expressed appreciation for Rotary's offer of vaccine but often countered

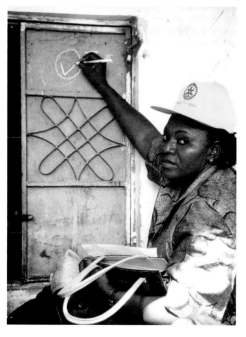

A chalk mark indicates that the children within have received polio vaccine. Rotarians join thousands of volunteer teams in house-to-house visits.

with appeals that Rotary might substitute some oral polio vaccine funds for the purchase of refrigerators, four-wheel drive vehicles, or other vaccines. UNICEF personnel, in particular, helped task force members hold firm to polio vaccine-only grants by reallocating some national UNICEF funds to

meet such requests.
As for Rotary's offer
of volunteer help,
ministers adopted a
wait-and-see attitude.
Pigman and his team
advised Rotarians
to start by choosing
an immunization
task within their
capacity, do it well,
and subordinate
their own desire for
publicity so as to
keep the limelight on
the health ministry
and its workers. Only in this way could Rotary, the "new kid on the block,"
gain their trust and confidence.

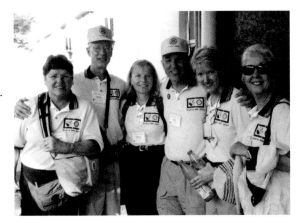

Hundreds of Rotarians, including these U.S. volunteers,
travel overseas to polio-endemic countries to help in
National Immunization Days. Their energy inspires their host
Rotarians as well as local health workers.

As reports of successful mass polio-immunization campaigns, particularly
those in the Americas, began to circulate in global health conferences, more
and more countries began to appreciate that polio could serve as the point of
the arrow in the EPI attack on childhood infectious diseases. In the minds of
many parents, polio was the most dreaded of all the diseases. The death of a
child from any infectious disease brought grief, yes. But a child paralyzed by
polio — a son reduced to a lifetime of begging, a daughter unmarriageable
— could be a crushing burden on a family already in marginal circumstances.

Thus the polio program began to draw people into the public health network. For some, polio immunization campaigns provided their first contact with a health provider. Baby censuses were conducted. Parents were urged to learn more about breastfeeding, oral rehydration, child-growth monitoring, vitamin A, and the importance of other vaccines. The morale of health workers, who were often poorly paid and underappreciated in developing nations, received a decided boost. They welcomed the interest and support of Rotarians and others volunteering to immunize children against polio.

By 1989, Rotary had approved grants for oral polio vaccine to 84 countries. Manuals outlined for Rotarians how their business knowledge and resources could help alleviate problems in areas of cold chain, communication, transportation, and mobilization of public acceptance of immunization. The seeds for national PolioPlus task forces were planted. With the initial spadework completed, and Rotary's ability to meet its $120 million pledge assured, the Rotary Immunization Task Force was disbanded in 1989. Rotary's fundraising campaign of the mid-1980s, however, had raised $247 million. Interest earned on unspent funds had further increased the PolioPlus pot. How were these additional resources to be used most effectively?

In the next four years, the Foundation Trustees found themselves bombarded with proposals: measles vaccine, cold-chain equipment, social mobilization tools, vaccine research, and expert personnel. Given that money for public health receives a tragically low percentage of national budgets, all such proposals represented urgent and valid needs. In 1994, to help with prioritizing these proposals, the Trustees created the International PolioPlus Committee (IPPC), an advisory body for the PolioPlus program.

Bill Sergeant, Foundation trustee and past RI vice president, was asked to lead the committee and determine the best use of remaining PolioPlus funds.

To ensure good communication with the RI Board and the Trustees, its 11-person membership provided for inclusion of four trustees and an RI director. Sergeant plunged into his volunteer assignment full-time, drafting strategic and tactical plans, counseling staff, and determining priorities. Sensing program fatigue, the IPPC advised the Trustees and Board of Directors to renew the commitment to PolioPlus through a resolution to the 1995 Council on Legislation. The resolution, affirming and endorsing the polio eradication goal as a "priority of the highest order" for Rotary International, passed unanimously.

Over the next 10 years, under Sergeant's guidance, the IPPC developed working procedures and terms of reference for regional and national PolioPlus committees. Sergeant sought advice from the U.S. Centers for Disease Control and Prevention and others concerning the geographic and program priorities for remaining PolioPlus funds. A spending plan ensured Rotary's ability to make grants over the long term (see page 100, "PolioPlus Grants").

Representatives of the spearheading partners of the Global Polio Eradication Initiative were invited to every IPPC meeting to update members on global issues and provide counsel on grant proposals. The committee established procedures enabling Rotary to respond rapidly to emergency needs. For instance, when strife-torn Sudan declared a cease-fire in 1997 to permit polio immunization, $400,000 was needed to charter aircraft to fly in the vaccine. Rotary responded in a matter of days with the money.

Every new PolioPlus grant now came with the condition that the recipient government or agency publicize it, helping to reduce objections from Rotarians that news media coverage too often ignored Rotary's role in polio eradication. High-level RI representatives dispatched to global health conferences, NID inaugurations, and meetings of intercountry coordinating agencies further raised Rotary's international profile. Internally, a program of awards was inaugurated to recognize Rotarians who provide outstanding service to PolioPlus.

Supplementing PolioPlus grants, the PolioPlus Partners program encouraged 7,000 clubs in hundreds of Rotary districts to help countries of their choice with surveillance tools and social mobilization needs, such as caps, T-shirts, vests, and posters. The value of their contributions, including matching funds from the World Fund of The Rotary Foundation, surpassed $33 million.

Under the steady hand of Sergeant and the IPPC, Rotary cemented its position as the leading private-sector partner in the Global Polio Eradication Initiative. Four spearheading partners were now shaping the course of the program: WHO served as the chief architect and strategist. UNICEF provided experience in training, social mobilization, and vaccine procurement. The CDC supplied technical support to laboratories and deployed experts in epidemiology and program management. Rotary provided money, volunteer muscle, and moral leadership. But the partners would soon turn to Rotary for an additional and most critical role.

From the outset of Rotary's involvement, it was apparent that PolioPlus funds alone could not meet the donor resource requirements of the Global Polio Eradication Initiative. Now the war was moving to more difficult battlefronts: developing countries with decrepit public-health infrastructures, weak or nonexistent surveillance systems, and limited national budgets. For some of these countries, the money for polio eradication would have to come entirely from the outside. But what was the price tag?

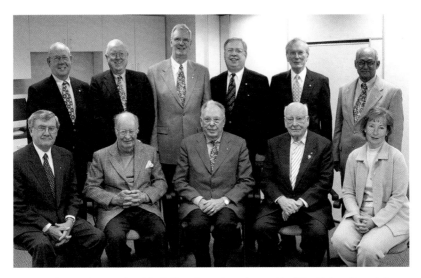

Since 1994, the International PolioPlus Committee has guided The Rotary Foundation Trustees on strategy and operations of Rotary's polio program. Serving in 2004-05 are (back row, from left) Ray Klinginsmith, Jim Lacy, Robert Scott, Ken Morgan, John Sever, Kaylan Banerjee, (front row) Vice Chair Herbert Pigman, Carlos Canseco, Trustee Chair Carlo Ravizza, Chair Bill Sergeant, and PolioPlus Division Manager Carol Pandak. Not present for photo: Frank Devlyn.

In 1994, WHO's polio initiative coordinator, Dr. Harry Hull, constructed a financial estimate for the global polio eradication program, indicating that at least $500 million in *additional* donor resources would be required to keep the program operating until the year 2000, the WHO target date. But IPPC members were hardly prepared for the bombshell that accompanied the financial estimate: WHO didn't have the money, and it didn't know where it was going to come from. Once again, Rotary would rise to a challenge.

CHAPTER

BRIDGING THE FUNDING GAP

BRIDGING THE FUNDING GAP

THE $500 MILLION in donor resources needed to maintain the momentum of the polio eradication initiative would have to come primarily from the overseas development budgets of wealthy nations, as well as the private sector. For both sources, there was a financial incentive to support the program.

Governments of polio-free nations were spending millions of dollars to protect their newborns against the threat of imported polioviruses. In the United States alone, the costs exceeded $300 million each year. Eradication of the virus and cessation of immunization would save an estimated $1 billion a year worldwide. As for the private sector, history had shown that healthy kids are a key to growing economies. Lower rates of morbidity and mortality had led to lower birth rates, helping many developing nations transition to a market economy. Clearly, support

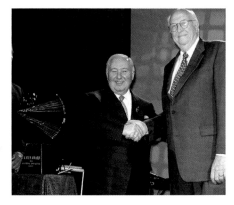

A $1 million award to The Rotary Foundation from the Bill & Melinda Gates Foundation, here accepted by Luis Giay from Bill Gates Sr., is one of many awards saluting Rotary's leadership in the polio eradication program. A complete list begins on page 102.

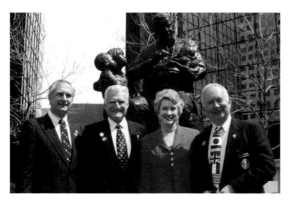

Sculptor Glenna Goodacre created the PolioPlus sculpture (above), now on public display in Denver, Evanston, and other cities. From left: Richard Gooding, whose firm cast the statue, Past RI President Herb Brown, Goodacre, and Grant Wilkins, who engaged the renowned artist's support of the program.

for creating more-robust public health systems would be in the self-interest of all.

But seeking special funding for polio eradication was a daunting task in a world where defense spending by governments outstrips development aid ($800 billion to $14 billion in 2002, according to a statement by World Bank president James Wolfensohn). In the shrinking foreign-aid environment of the last decade of the 20th century, many primary health care systems had deteriorated.

The idea of Rotary entering the arena of advocacy to governments was not only new; it was foreign to its traditions. Nevertheless, Sergeant and Sever attended a meeting in Washington, D.C., in December 1994 of a nascent coalition aimed at persuading the U.S. government to increase its financial support of polio eradication. Although the term *lobbying* evoked negative reactions in some minds, the need was critical. Problems with nomenclature were resolved by defining Rotary's role as that of an advocate with the stated purpose of "communicating to leaders at global, national, and local levels the benefits of the eradication of polio by the year 2000, so that the financial, technical, and other resources required to reach this goal will be committed on a timely basis."

Rotary soon found itself in the lead. In January 1995, Sever, on behalf of the new coalition (Rotary, the Task Force for Child Survival and Development, the U.S. Committee for UNICEF, and the U.S. Academy of Pediatrics), stated the case for polio eradication at a public-witness hearing of a U.S. House of Representatives appropriations subcommittee. Rotary engaged Capitol Associates, a Washington-based consulting firm experienced in health advocacy, to guide the U.S. strategy. Pigman (again serving as RI general secretary) was asked to chair the Polio Eradication Advocacy Task Force following his second retirement in June. His full-time volunteer assignment lasted four years. He drafted a global strategy targeting 30 potential donor nations. With the help of advocacy advisers, the task force members, often in concert with WHO and UNICEF colleagues, put the case for polio before heads of state, key legislators, and development aid ministers. Presentation tools were created, including a 16-page color brochure translated into 13 languages, and placed in the hands of parliamentarians of many donor nations.

In the United States, Rotary held annual congressional receptions to celebrate progress and salute the legislators who translated Rotary's appeals into funding. Sever and Pigman made frequent appearances before congressional committees. U.S. appropriations for polio eradication, funneled through the CDC and USAID, rose from a level of $9.8 million in 1995 to $133 million in 2004, a nine-year total exceeding $933 million.

Advocacy efforts brought increased support from Australia, Canada, Denmark, France, Germany, Japan, the Netherlands, Taiwan, the United

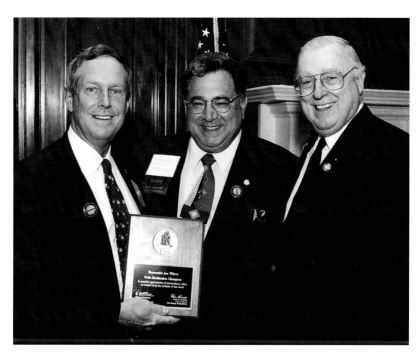

Rotary has helped to raise more than $1.7 billion in funds from donor nations. In the United States, an annual Rotary-sponsored reception honors key members of Congress with the Polio Eradication Champion Award (presented here to Representative Joe Wilson by Lou Picconi and Jim Lacy).

Kingdom, and other countries. Past RI vice presidents Robert Scott and Richard Slager, both medical doctors, assumed leadership of the task force. Rotary took the lead in forming the Polio Advocacy Group, through which the spearheading partners began to fully coordinate their fundraising efforts.

The advocacy program cost less than $3 million in PolioPlus funds, and it proved to be a good investment. By mid-2003, the joint advocacy efforts led by Rotary and its partners resulted in more than $1.5 billion in polio-specific grants from the public sector. Why did these advocacy efforts succeed? The idea of a public-private partnership resonated well with government leaders. The war on polio had a target date, a budget, a proven strategy, and an effective weapon in oral polio vaccine. It was enjoying spectacular progress. The list of polio-free nations increased steadily. The number of cases dropped 99.8 percent. And from a humanitarian standpoint, what better goal than a victory over the greatest crippler of children?

Despite the growing financial support of donor countries, however, the forecast expense of combating polio in poor countries began to exceed even the most optimistic funding projections. In 1998, the Trustees gave Pigman approval to explore a new source of support: the private sector, including foundations, corporations, and wealthy individuals. The search led to the newly established United Nations Foundation, funded with a $1 billion pledge from Ted Turner. Pigman

The United Nations Foundation, launched by Ted Turner, funded a joint Rotary-UN Foundation appeal to the global private sector that raised $112 million for polio. Here, past RI presidents Frank Devlyn (left) and Herb Brown (right) salute Turner and UN Secretary-General Kofi Annan.

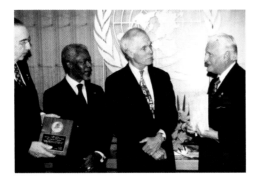

presented the UN Foundation with a $120 million proposal to improve polio surveillance systems in Africa.

Although the proposal was too ambitious, it opened the door. UN Foundation President Tim Wirth immediately perceived that the polio eradication initiative represented a model of the kind of partnerships his agency was hoping to create. Wirth and Pigman worked out a plan for a joint appeal to the private sector, to be funded by the UN Foundation and managed by Rotary.

The plan was approved in April 2000, and the newly formed Polio Eradication Private Sector Initiative Task Force, headed by Slager for Rotary and Steve Strickland for the UN Foundation, enlisted and trained 150 Rotarians worldwide to carry the message to corporate and foundation boardrooms. Dan Henry, Pigman, and Jack Blane successively directed the campaign, which raised $112 million, including a gift of $50 million from the Bill & Melinda Gates Foundation;

Following the 1988 resolution to eradicate polio, Rotary's $5.3 million grant to WHO funded a leadership team that jump-started the global program. Past RI President Bob Barth (left) confirmed Rotary's commitment to WHO Director-General Hiroshi Nakajima.

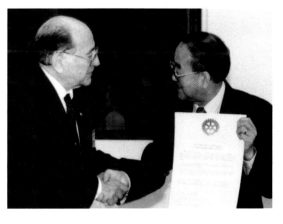

$29 million from the UN Foundation; $7.2 million (including some matching funds from the UN Foundation) from Trick or Treat for UNICEF, conducted by the U.S. Committee for UNICEF; and $1 million gifts from the Advantage Trust of Hong Kong, Pew Charitable Trusts, and Wyeth Laboratories.

Corporate contributions, however, did not reach expected levels. They were negatively affected by a global economic downturn that coincided with the period of the campaign, followed by a jolt to the business and philanthropic communities in the wake of the 11 September terrorist attacks in the United States. Nevertheless, a secondary purpose of the campaign was accomplished: Corporate leaders gained a better understanding and appreciation of Rotary, the UN Foundation, and each organization's purposes.

With expenses rising and donor requirements still unmet, Rotary was destined to step forward once again. The September 2000 polio summit in New York had brought together Wirth and Pigman with an officer of the World Bank, a leading lender of funds for public health in developing countries. They discussed how the polio program might tap into World Bank resources to accelerate the final stages of polio eradication. From a follow-up meeting in January 2001, attended by Slager, emerged an idea for the World Bank's International Development Association to offer low-interest loans to major polio-endemic countries for the purchase of oral polio vaccine. The appealing feature of the plan, subsequently forged by Rotary, the UN Foundation, the Gates Foundation, and the World Bank, was that such a loan could be immediately excused if a private-sector source would pay off the loan "up front," at 40 percent of its face value. The Gates Foundation pledged $25 million for such loans, provided they would be matched by Rotary or other private-sector sources. It was a good deal. In effect, a Rotary contribution of

$1 would be matched by $1 from the Gates Foundation, which in turn would trigger an equivalent contribution of $3 from the World Bank.

There was, however, a problem. Rotary didn't have $25 million in available PolioPlus funds to match the Gates Foundation offer. In October 2001, Rotary Foundation Trustee and Past RI President Jim Lacy proposed to the Trustees that Rotary launch a new polio fundraising campaign among Rotarians. The Trustees and the RI Board of Directors concurred, convinced that Rotarians would react positively. More than 50 percent of members had joined the organization since the campaign of the mid-1980s, and thousands of these members were women. All these new members would welcome a chance to participate in a program that held a number-one priority in their organization. The goal of the one-year campaign, named Fulfilling Our Promise: Eradicate Polio, was set at $80 million, sufficient not only to meet the Gates Foundation-World Bank challenge but also to replenish the dwindling coffers of the PolioPlus Fund.

Trustee Chair and Past RI President Luis Giay chaired the new International Polio Eradication Fundraising Campaign Committee. Pigman was named campaign

In their second global fundraising effort, Rotarians once again came up with creative ways to raise funds, such as a snow sculpture contest in Winnipeg, Manitoba, Canada. The one-year campaign raised more than $130 million.

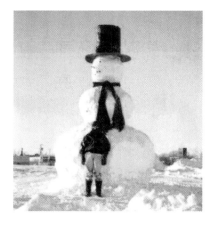

director, and John Osterlund (later named as general manager of The Rotary Foundation) was tapped as associate director. In the five months preceding the campaign launch on 1 July 2002, leaders of 43 national or multinational committees were selected and trained in a series of global seminars, videotapes and printed materials were developed, and district and regional training sessions were conducted for some 4,000 area coordinators.

Rotarians worldwide dug into their own pockets and once again unleashed creative fundraising efforts involving the public. Scott assumed the leadership of the campaign in October 2002; nine months later at the RI Convention in Brisbane, Australia, Trustee Chair Glen Kinross and RI President Bhichai Rattakul announced that the campaign had reached $88.5 million in cash, pledges, commitments, and District Designated Fund allocations. By late 2004, the total surpassed $130 million. Rotary had once again demonstrated its commitment.

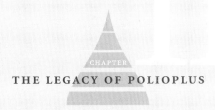

CHAPTER 11

THE LEGACY OF POLIOPLUS

THE LEGACY OF POLIOPLUS

As a result of the efforts of Rotary International and its Foundation and those of its partners, more than two billion children have received oral polio vaccine since 1985. Five million people, mainly in the developing world, who otherwise would have been paralyzed, are walking today because they have been immunized against polio; 500,000 cases continue to be prevented each year.

Apart from these humanitarian achievements, PolioPlus has had a significant impact in other areas. It has altered the public's perception of Rotary. Among leaders in government, business, and philanthropy, PolioPlus has awakened a new appreciation for the power of partnerships in the quest to improve the human condition.

Addressing the 2001 RI Convention in San Antonio, Texas, USA, Dr. Gro Harlem Brundtland, who was then director-general of WHO, praised Rotary's support. "You were the first with the vision to deliver polio vaccine to every child," she said, "and you took action to make it happen." Carol Bellamy, executive director of UNICEF, said: "The volunteerism exemplified by Rotary International is an engine for renewal and change in every society. And it is that same volunteer spirit, rooted in compassion and a profound sense of responsibility to our fellow human beings, that offers so much hope for the future."

This change in the public's perception has also had a significant impact on Rotary itself.

"Two things have happened as a result of PolioPlus," remarks Past RI Director Kalyan Banerjee, of India. "Governments have discovered Rotary, and Rotarians have discovered themselves."

Throughout the world, national and local press, radio, and television reported the leadership and participation of Rotarians in polio eradication. George Tsaka, chair of Malawi's National PolioPlus Committee, says: "[The image of Rotary] among the general public now is that of rescuer, provider, a friend [to those] in need. The list is endless."

His assessment echoes the view of scores of other Rotarians who have personally witnessed the impact of the PolioPlus program on the public's view of Rotary. This growing understanding and appreciation of Rotary's purpose came at a propitious period in its history. As the last century ended and the new one began, membership in many service clubs, labor unions, and other civil society organizations stagnated or declined. PolioPlus helped Rotary maintain, and even increase, its membership. Rotary's profile in Turkey, for example, rapidly changed when Rotary clubs there joined the country's drive against polio. From 1955 to 1985, Rotary in Turkey had slowly grown to a level of 43 clubs. With the launch of PolioPlus, Turkish Rotarians began to get appeals from communities wanting to start Rotary clubs. Rotary in Turkey grew fourfold. Today, the country has 213 Rotary clubs with more than 7,000 members. Similarly, Indonesia had only 21 Rotary clubs in 1985; today, it has 87.

These changes in public attitude were welcome indeed, especially in Asian and African countries that had gained independence in the last four decades of the 20th century. In most of these new nations, Rotary was an idea imported during colonial rule, and expatriates dominated club membership. Leaders of the newly independent governments harbored suspicions about Rotary, and public perceptions were less than flattering.

"Despite decades of Rotary service, Rotary and 'Roti' had become synonymous," reflects India's National PolioPlus Committee Chair Deepak Kapur. "*Roti* means 'bread' in the Hindi language, and Rotary clubs had become known as Roti clubs, places where the rich congregated to eat and drink, to make merry. The clubs were doing excellent work. They fed the hungry, clothed the naked, and sheltered the homeless. But the perception continued. That is, until Rotary decided on the PolioPlus program. Suddenly, perceptions started changing. Rotary underwent the Cinderella-to-princess transformation. It gained credibility, acceptability, and respect."

There is little question that PolioPlus has helped to solidify Rotary's position as an indigenous force for good in the societies of scores of newly independent nations. "They have come to see the true face of the organization and to consider it as a major partner in the fight against disease, poverty, ignorance, [and] illiteracy and a partner in the development of mankind," concludes Antoine Muyombano, chair of Rwanda's National PolioPlus Committee.

PolioPlus has affected Rotarians as individuals. Playing a role in a significant cause fulfills a basic human need. Whether as contributors, vaccinators, or both, Rotarians have taken enormous pride in their collective achievement. The participation of spouses and children in PolioPlus has nurtured the idea that Rotary can also be a family affair. Through PolioPlus, Rotarians have formed bonds with hundreds of thousands of young adults and leaders in Interact and Rotaract clubs.

PolioPlus has contributed to a greater sense of unity in Rotary, globally and within nations. In Nigeria, reports National PolioPlus Committee Chair

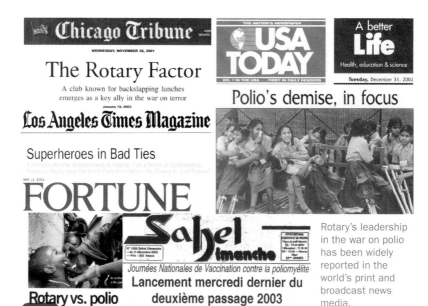

Chicago Tribune

WEDNESDAY, NOVEMBER 28, 2001

The Rotary Factor

A club known for backslapping lunches
emerges as a key ally in the war on terror

January 19, 2003

Los Angeles Times Magazine

Superheroes in Bad Ties

A Precious Window of Opportunity Is Closing. Can a Bunch of Glad-Handing
Rotarians Really Save the World From Polio before the Chance Is Lost Forever?

MAR 12, 2003

FORTUNE

Rotary vs. polio

THE NATION'S NEWSPAPER

USA TODAY

NO. 1 IN THE USA . . . FIRST IN DAILY READERS

A better
Life

Health, education & science

Tuesday, December 31, 2002

Polio's demise, in focus

Sahel dimanche

OFFICE NATIONAL
D'EDITION ET DE PRESSE
Place du petit Marché
Tél. : 73-24-86/87
Télécopieur : 73 90 90
B.P. 12618 — Niamey
Niger

N° 1058 Sahel Dimanche
du 5 décembre 2003
Prix : 250 francs

12ème ANNÉE

Journées Nationales de Vaccination contre la poliomyélite

**Lancement mercredi dernier du
deuxième passage 2003**

Rotary's leadership
in the war on polio
has been widely
reported in the
world's print and
broadcast news
media.

Adedehin Ebunolu Adefeso, "Rotarians have been united in a common cause,
cutting across the country's divergent ethnic, language, and cultural groupings."

For Rotary International, the horizons of service were expanded.
PolioPlus demonstrated the collective strength of its members. Resolution
23-34 was retired to a respectful place in Rotary's history. In its place emerged
a realization that the yoke of Rotary service can easily balance service to the
local community with service to the world community. And this portends for
Rotary a bright future and enduring place in society.

Ideally, this brief history of PolioPlus would conclude with an epilogue bearing the triumphant news that somewhere, perhaps in a remote village in Africa, a health worker has found and confirmed the last case of polio. That is not possible. As of mid-2004, major battles were still underway in two areas where the virus persists. India had five national and two subnational days of immunization scheduled for 2004, Nigeria and surrounding countries targeted 250 million children in synchronized campaigns, and all six remaining polio-endemic countries were resolved to find the last case in 2004.

The *Global Polio Eradication Initiative Strategic Plan 2004-2008*, developed by WHO, UNICEF, CDC, and Rotary, is guiding the final stages of the war on polio. Donor nations continue their financial support, and the bonds among the four spearheading partners remain strong.

Rotary has stated clearly that it is in the war for the duration. The Trustees and the RI Board have agreed that the goal of PolioPlus is the global certification of polio eradication, eradication being the interruption of the transmission of the wild poliovirus. An independent global commission will consider global certification of the eradication of polio when no wild poliovirus cases have occurred for at least three years in the presence of certification-standard surveillance, and when all wild poliomyelitis vaccine stocks have been appropriately contained.

Meanwhile, the legacy of Rotary's first global service program continues to grow. Twenty years ago, the dream of a polio-free world was a distant star. Today, it is within reach.

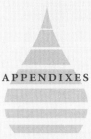

APPENDIXES

POLIOPLUS GRANTS

1979-2004 (30 June)

Country	Total (US$)
Afghanistan	7,862,028
Algeria	1,025,184
Angola	5,637,426
Antigua and Barbuda	5,443
Argentina	2,153,709
Armenia – MECACAR*	130,924
Azerbaijan – MECACAR*	223,720
Bangladesh	16,302,084
Belize	66,408
Benin	1,705,655
Bolivia	1,357,307
Botswana	360,000
Brazil	6,076,620
Bulgaria	239,448
Burkina Faso	1,652,984
Burundi	479,635
Cambodia	300,000
Cameroun	1,053,009
Cape Verde	105,000
Central African Republic	832,699
Chad	1,434,784
Chile	665,103
China	22,126,748
Colombia	3,043,511
Comoros Islands	44,352
Congo Republic	1,224,193
Costa Rica	203,700

Country	Total (US$)
Côte d'Ivoire	2,942,952
Cuba	547,015
Democratic Republic of the Congo**	11,677,312
Dominican Republic	596,969
Ecuador	1,314,088
Egypt	3,333,999
El Salvador	1,267,479
Equatorial Guinea	84,000
Ethiopia	5,662,716
Gabon	176,926
Gambia	289,353
Georgia	92,168
Ghana	2,605,524
Grenada	9,925
Guatemala	1,896,536
Guinea	901,508
Guinea-Bissau	294,501
Guyana	96,357
Haiti	1,533,229
Honduras	1,436,795
India	51,412,116
Indonesia	13,050,558
Iraq	457,916
Jamaica	94,788
Jordan	416,958
Kazakhstan – MECACAR*	455,229

* Operation MECACAR
** Total includes grants for Zaire.

Country	Total (US$)
Kenya	2,852,207
Korea	226,000
Kyrgyzstan – MECACAR*	144,609
Laos	280,671
Lebanon	336,314
Lesotho	139,981
Liberia	514,855
Madagascar	1,952,152
Malawi	1,323,253
Mali	1,264,782
Mauritania	495,770
Mauritius	34,773
Mexico	9,223,600
Moldova	55,687
Morocco	2,420,037
Myanmar	7,004,071
Namibia	155,820
Nepal	5,619,013
Nicaragua	1,064,485
Niger	2,810,518
Nigeria	32,600,781
Oman	178,848
Pakistan	21,222,550
Panama	652,251
Papua New Guinea	322,001
Paraguay	652,097
Peru	3,265,120
Philippines	6,714,046
Romania	792,720
Rwanda	938,753
São Tomé e Príncipe	84,000
Senegal	556,668
Sierra Leone	644,797

Country	Total (US$)
Solomon Islands	6,250
Somalia	6,123,695
South Africa	43,944
Sri Lanka	2,276,059
St. Lucia	60,607
St. Vincent and the Grenadines	11,073
Sudan	8,700,210
Suriname	9,063
Swaziland	63,200
Tajikistan	76,865
Tajikistan – MECACAR*	467,060
Tanzania	2,592,122
Thailand	2,566,792
Togo	918,563
Trinidad and Tobago	60,758
Tunisia	555,891
Turkey	5,658,227
Turkey – MECACAR*	3,783,731
Turkmenistan	48,281
Turkmenistan – MECACAR*	258,446
Uganda	2,762,170
Ukraine	105,944
Uruguay	227,292
Uzbekistan	332,444
Uzbekistan – MECACAR*	883,159
Venezuela	850,266
Vietnam	3,602,772
Yemen	1,231,370
Yugoslavia	298,834
Zambia	964,194
Zimbabwe	1,741,448
Regional and other grants	117,363,309
Total	$450,145,860

RECOGNITIONS AND HONORS

Conferred upon Rotary International, The Rotary Foundation,
and Rotarians in Recognition of PolioPlus

Year	Conferring Body/Individual Award/Honor Recipient/Honoree	Notes
1985	**UNICEF** **Plaque of appreciation** **Rotary International**	Presented by UNICEF Executive Director James Grant and received by RI President-elect M.A.T. Caparas
1985	**Turkish Ministry of Health and Social Assistance** **Plaque of appreciation** **Rotary International**	Presented by Turkish Minister of Health and Social Assistance Mehmet Aydin and received by RI President-elect M.A.T. Caparas
1987	**Government of Peru** **Daniel Alcides Carrion Award** **Rotary International**	In recognition of RI's efforts in support of Peru's Expanded Program on Immunization; Peru's highest honor in the field of health and medicine
1987	**American Association of World Health** **World Health Day Award** **Rotary International**	In recognition of Rotary's "outstanding commitment to the eradication of polio in the Americas and to universal child immunization by 1990"
1987	**National Conference of Christians and Jews** **Silver Medallion Brotherhood Award** **Past RI President Herbert G. Brown**	For his "tireless efforts to extend the helping hands of brotherhood not only in his home community of Clearwater (Florida, USA) but internationally through his work with Rotary's PolioPlus Campaign"

Year	Conferring Body/Individual Award/Honor Recipient/Honoree	Notes
1988	**UNICEF** **International Child Survival Award** **Rotary International**	In recognition of the PolioPlus program as a "significant contribution to the advancement of child survival"; inaugural year of award
1988	**American Academy of Pediatrics** **Presidential Certificate for Outstanding Service** **Rotary International**	Highest award given by the APA, a 37,000-member organization of pediatricians in the United States, Canada, and Latin America
1989	**Government of Venezuela** **Dr. Enrique Tejera Medal of Health** **Rotary International**	Award named for former Venezuelan health minister
1989	**Government of Venezuela** **National Medal of Health** **The Rotary Foundation**	
1989	**National Society of Fund-Raising Executives of the United States** **Outstanding Philanthropic Organization Award** **Rotary International**	Regarded as most prestigious award in U.S. philanthrophy
1989	**National Council for International Health** **Award for Organizations in International Health** **Rotary International**	U.S.-based nonprofit organization now known as Global Health Council

Year	Conferring Body/Individual / Award/Honor / Recipient/Honoree	Notes
1989	**UNICEF-Canada** **Award of recognition** **Rotary International**	For Rotary's "outstanding contribution to the immunization decade" through PolioPlus and specifically the efforts of Canada's PolioPlus Campaign Committee
1989	**U.S. President George Bush** **President's Volunteer Action Award** **Walter Maddocks**	In recognition of his efforts as executive director of the PolioPlus Campaign
1990	**UNICEF** **Medal of recognition** **Rotary International**	For its efforts in promoting and organizing three NIDs for India, Nepal, and Sri Lanka; presented by UNICEF Executive Director James Grant and accepted on behalf of Rotary by Past RI Director Manohar Manchanda, Rotary Immunization Task Force chair
1990	**California Medical Association** **Plaque** **Rotary International**	CMA President Dr. Charles W. Plows called PolioPlus "a shining example of the great strides that can be made in alleviating human suffering through preventative medicine."
1990	**U.S. Agency for International Development** **Letter of recognition** **Rotary International**	USAID, in its fifth annual report to Congress on its child survival program, highlighted both the PolioPlus fundraising campaign and the work of PolioPlus volunteers; Dr. John Sever accepted the letter on RI's behalf.
1990	**Honduran Ministry of Education** **José Cecilio Del Valle National Science Award** **Dr. Romón Alcero Castro**	In recognition of his PolioPlus efforts

Year	Conferring Body/Individual Award/Honor Recipient/Honoree	Notes
1991	**Venezuelan Ministry of Health** **Health Medal** **RI President Paulo V.C. Costa**	Awarded by Minister of Health Dr. Manuel Adrianza
1991	**Government of Ecuador** **Public health award** **RI President Paulo V.C. Costa**	In appreciation of his work on behalf of the PolioPlus Campaign; Ecuador's highest public health award
1991	**Queen Elizabeth II** **Member of the Most Excellent Order of the British Empire** **RI Director Roy Whitby**	In recognition of his work as chair of the United Kingdom, Ireland, and Gibraltar PolioPlus Committee, which raised more than £9 million (US$16 million)
1991	**Government of Brazil** **Oswaldo Cruz gold medal** **RI President Paulo V.C. Costa**	Presented by Brazilian Minister of Health Alceni Guerra, in recognition of Rotary's worldwide PolioPlus Campaign
1991	**City of Medicine (Durham, North Carolina, USA) Awards Program** **City of Medicine Award** **Rotary International**	Presented annually to individuals and organizations who "have made extraordinary contributions to medicine in the public interest"; accepted by Past RI President and Rotary Foundation Trustee Chair Carlos Canseco; first organization to receive the award
1992	**U.S. Centers for Disease Control and Prevention** **Auxiliary Mission Support Award** **Rotary International**	In recognition of Rotary's worldwide support through PolioPlus of the Expanded Programme on Immunization, as well as the U.S. Rotary clubs' focus on domestic immunization projects

Year	Conferring Body/Individual Award/Honor Recipient/Honoree	Notes
1992	**Rehabilitation International** **Citation of Merit** **Rotary International**	Presented by Dr. Fenmore Seton, president of Rehabilitation International, and accepted on behalf of Rotary by Past District Governor Yusuf Kodwavwala
1992	**American Institute for Public Service** **Jefferson Award** **Leslie S. Wright**	Selected as local winner (Alabama, USA) of community service award for his "voluntarism in worldwide polio immunization efforts" as International PolioPlus Campaign Committee chair
1993	**World Health Organization** **Health-for-All Gold Medal** **Rotary International**	WHO's highest honor
1993	**Bolivian Ministry of Health** **Special citation** **Bolivia's National PolioPlus Committee**	For its efforts in attaining high levels of immunization coverage
1993	**Colombian Ministry of Health** **Jorge Bejerano Health and Social Service Award** **Dr. Alberto Delgadillo Vargas**	For his contribution to the health of the Colombian people; most prestigious honor of its kind in Colombia
1993	**Venezuelan Ministry of Health** **National Health Cross** **Dr. Lisandro Lattuf**	For his "selfless dedication to the campaign to eradicate polio" as chair of Venezuela's National PolioPlus Committee
1994	**Government of the Philippines** **Plaque of recognition** **The Rotary Foundation**	For its participation in the 1993 NIDs, in which more than 9.6 million children were vaccinated; presented by Philippine President Fidel V. Ramos

Year	Conferring Body/Individual	Notes
	Award/Honor	
	Recipient/Honoree	
1994	**Mexico's National Immunization Advisory Board**	For its generous contribution to Mexico's polio eradication program
	Diploma	
	The Rotary Foundation	
1995	**UNICEF**	In honor of RI's PolioPlus program, which to date had immunized more than 600 million children against polio; first time award, which recognizes "individuals whose actions have resulted in a meaningful benefit to children," given to an organization
	Audrey Hepburn Child Advocate Award	
	Rotary International	
1995	**World Health Organization**	In recognition of his work as chair of Peru's National PolioPlus Committee; presented on 7 April, World Health Day, at Pan American Health Organization headquarters in Washington, D.C.
	Macedo Award	
	RI Director Gustavo Gross	
1996	**City of Juarez, Mexico**	10.7-meter (35-foot) blue-and-gold Rotary wheel with a statue of Canseco at its center; erected in median of Avenida de Las Americas, the busy thoroughfare leading to the U.S. border; nearby plaza renamed Plaza Rotaria
	Monument ("World Without Polio")	
	Rotary International and Past RI President Carlos Canseco	
1996	**National Council for International Health**	One of four awarded annually; Rotary's "outstanding leadership and progress toward the eradication of polio" hailed by NCIH President Frank Lostumbo as example of "how the private sector can support international health"
	Leadership in Global Health	
	Rotary International	

Year	Conferring Body/Individual Award/Honor Recipient/Honoree	Notes
1996	**Government of Angola** **Statue** **Rotary International (along with WHO, UNICEF, and Angolan Ministry of Health)**	In recognition of their efforts in supporting Angola's historic polio immunization effort; unveiled by Angolan President José Eduardo dos Santos
1996	**Angolan Ministry of Health** **Statuette** **Rotary International**	For its support of Angola's first-ever NIDs, held in August and September; presented by Acting Minister of Health Teresa Cohen and accepted on Rotary's behalf by Rotary Foundation Trustee Tony Serrano
1996	**Republic of Namibia** **Ministry of Health and Social Services Certificate** **Rotary International**	For its contribution to Namibia's NIDs
1996	**Venezuelan Ministry of Health and Social Welfare** **Plaque** **Rotary International, The Rotary Foundation, Venezuelan Rotarians**	In recognition of their efforts, through the PolioPlus Campaign, to stop the spread of the poliovirus in Venezuela
1996	**Children's Vaccine Initiative** **Jenner Award** **The Rotary Foundation**	Inaugural year of award; CVI cosponsors: WHO, UNICEF, UN Development Programme, World Bank, and Rockefeller Foundation
1998	**U.S. Centers for Disease Control and Prevention** **Champion of Prevention** **Rotary International**	In recognition of Rotary's work in the global initiative to eradicate polio; presented by CDC Acting Director Claire Broome

Year	Conferring Body/Individual Award/Honor Recipient/Honoree	Notes
1998	**World Health Organization** **50th Anniversary Award** **Rotary International**	In honor of its contributions to polio eradication efforts in Africa
1998	**World of Children** **Kellogg's Hannah Neil World of Children Award** **Past RI Vice President Bill Sergeant**	In recognition of his work as chair of the International PolioPlus Committee; major international award that recognizes those who make a world of difference in the lives of children across the globe
1999	**International Public Relations Association** **President's Award** **Rotary International**	Honors an individual or organization for "outstanding contributions to better world understanding"
2000	**Kentucky State (USA) House of Representatives and Senate** **Citations** **Rotary International and the Rotary Club of Frankfort, Kentucky**	For their work in combating polio
2000	**American Medical Association** **Outstanding Global Health Initiative Award** **Global Polio Eradication Initiative (including Rotary International)**	Award honors physicians and health initiatives that further health information and medical practice worldwide; accepted by RI President Carlo Ravizza on behalf of Rotary International and other spearheading partners (WHO, CDC, and UNICEF)

Year	Conferring Body/Individual Award/Honor Recipient/Honoree	Notes
2000	**Metro Manila (Philippines) Department of Health Center for Health Development**	For its generous support, active participation, and effective mobilization of all sectoral groups in successfully attaining a polio-free Philippines in the year 2000
	Certificate of appreciation	
	Rotary International	
2002	**Bill & Melinda Gates Foundation**	In recognition of Rotary's leadership and impact in the field of public health, most notably the organization's top priority of eradicating polio; recognition carries with it $1 million award
	Gates Award for Global Health	
	The Rotary Foundation	
2002	**Pan American Health Organization**	For his invaluable contributions to public health in the Americas
	Public Health Hero of the Americas	
	Past RI President Carlos Canseco	
2003	**Iowa (USA) Orthopaedic Society**	Award carried with it $5,000 contribution to Rotary's polio eradication fundraising campaign
	James J. Puhl, MD, Humanitarian Award	
	The Rotary Foundation	
2004	**American Academy of Pediatrics**	Presented by AAP Immediate Past President Dr. E. Stephen Edwards and accepted by RI President Jonathan Majiyagbe on Rotary's behalf
	Excellence in Public Service Award	
	Rotary International